Cookbook for Beginners

Easy & Delicious Lunch Recipes

Copyright 2020 by Jerryk luna - All rights reserved

Table of Contents

Introduction

First and foremost, I want to give a huge thank you for purchasing my book, *'Cookbook for Beginners: Easy & Delicious Lunch Ideas & Lunch Recipes'*

I hope you are prepared to experience one of the most wonderful cooking in the world from the comfort of your own kitchen.

In this book you will learn about the easy & delicious lunch recipes from many countries. I am collecting the best lunch recipes from Brazil, Jamaica, Ethiopia, German, Mexico & Italy. All recipe with necessary kitchen equipment.

A food that is rich in both its flavors and colors.

Combined with local vegetation and amazing local herbs and spices, with traditional procedure. Incorporating some of the oldest cooking techniques on the planet, it consists of the heartiest of stews, some of the richest seafood dishes in the world, and of course the most decadent of deserts.

It offers more than enough to get you and your family through the Delicious Lunch Ideas & Lunch Recipes – so what are you waiting for? Dive on in and get exploring!

Servings: 3

Ingredients:

- ½ table-spoon cooking oil
- 1 small yellow onion, chopped
- 1 cup dry pinto beans, dried
- Freshly cracked pepper to taste
- 7.5 ounces canned diced tomatoes
- 2 ounces dry Spanish chorizo, diced
- 2 cloves garlic, minced
- 1 bay leaf
- 1½ cups low sodium chicken broth

Method:

1. Select 'Sauté' button and press 'Adjust' button once. Add chorizo and cook until it is slightly crisp on the edges.
2. Add onion and garlic and cook until onions are translucent.
3. Add beans, pepper and bay leaf and stir. Pour broth and stir.
4. Close the lid. Select 'Beans/Chili' button and set the timer for 32 minutes.
5. Remove the bay leaf. Add tomatoes and stir.
6. Select 'Sauté' button and press 'Adjust' button twice. Let it simmer until thick.
7. Serving options: Rice, tortillas, tortilla chips or any other toppings of your choice.

Servings: 8

Ingredients

<u>For jerk prawns:</u>

- 1 large onion, minced
- 12 cloves garlic, minced
- 9-10 scotch bonnet chilies or more to taste
- 1 tea-spoon ground nutmeg
- ½ tea-spoon ground cinnamon
- 4 tea-spoons whole pimento
- ½ cup vegetable oil
- ½ cup water
- 2 tea-spoons salt
- ½ cup spring onions, chopped
- 2 table-spoons ginger, minced
- 4 tea-spoons fresh thyme
- 10 whole cloves
- 2 table-spoons brown sugar
- 6 bay leaves
- ½ cup vinegar
- ½ tea-spoon black pepper
- 4 pounds prawns

<u>For coconut Callaloo rice:</u>

- 12 stalks callaloo, discard stems, roughly chop the leaves
- 6 cloves garlic, minced
- 2 whole green scotch bonnet
- 6 table-spoons butter
- Salt to taste
- Pepper to taste
- 8 cups coconut milk
- 6 sprigs thyme
- 4 spring onions, finely chopped
- 2 pounds basmati rice

- Sautéed vegetables to serve

Method:

1. To make jerk prawns: Add all the ingredients of jerk prawns except prawns into a food processor or blender and blend until smooth.
2. Place prawns in a bowl. Pour the mixture over it. Coat the prawns well. Let it marinate for a while.
3. Set an outdoor grill or BBQ to preheat over medium heat setting.
4. Meanwhile, make the callaloo rice as follows: Pour coconut milk in a large saucepan.
5. Place the saucepan over medium heat. When it begins to simmer, add callaloo.
6. When it begins to boil, add thyme, bonnet peppers, spring onions, thyme and garlic and mix well. Let it simmer for 12 minutes.
7. Stir in the rice and butter.
8. Lower heat and cover with a lid. Cook until rice is al dente.
9. Brush oil over the grill grates. Place prawns on the preheated grill. Cook for 3-4 minutes. Flip sides and cook the other side for 3-4 minutes. Baste with the marinade while grilling.
10. Serve rice over individual serving plates. Place prawns over it. Serve with sautéed vegetables of your choice.

Servings: 4

Ingredients:

- 3 ounces wild garlic ramps
- 3 table-spoons grated parmesan cheese
- 1/4 cup rapeseed oil or canola oil (cold-pressed)
- 2 table-spoons pine nuts
- Salt and pepper, to taste

Method:

1. Rinse the wild garlic ramps thoroughly under running water. Drain them well and chop coarsely.
2. Take a food processor and place the chopped wild garlic ramps, cheese, rapeseed oil and pine nuts into it.
3. Pulse for 50 seconds until the mixture becomes a smooth paste.
4. Transfer to a bowl and season it with pepper and salt.
5. Mix it with a spoon and serve!

Servings: 4

Ingredients:

- ¼ cup olive oil
- 2 cloves garlic, chopped
- 2 stalks celery, chopped
- 3 eggs
- ½ cup fresh parsley, chopped
- 7.5 ounces canned diced tomatoes with its liquid
- Red pepper flakes to taste
- ¾ cup red wine
- 1 onion, chopped
- 1-pound ground beef
- ½ green bell pepper, chopped
- ¾ cup red wine

Method:

1. Select 'Sauté' button. Add oil. When the oil heated, add onion and sauté until golden brown.
2. Add beef, eggs, tomatoes, celery, bell pepper and parsley into a bowl and mix well.
3. Transfer into the instant pot. Cook until beef is brown. Press 'Cancel' button.
4. Close the lid. Select 'Slow cook' button and set the timer for 1 hour.
5. Add red wine vinegar and red pepper flakes after about 25-30 minutes of cooking.

Servings: 6-8

Ingredients

- 6-8 pieces chicken

<u>For seasoning:</u>

- 2 tea-spoons black pepper powder
- 2 tea-spoons Maggie chicken seasoning
- 2 tea-spoons paprika
- 2 tea-spoons Island jerk seasoning
- 2 tea-spoons paprika
- 2 tea-spoons salt
- 2 tea-spoons Maggie all-purpose
- 2 tea-spoons cayenne pepper

<u>Other ingredients:</u>

- 2 stalks scallions, chopped
- 2 table-spoons ketchup
- ½ cup vegetable oil or more if required
- A little water
- 1 hot pepper, sliced
- 2 cloves garlic, crushed
- 2 sprigs thyme, chopped
- 2 tomatoes, sliced
- 2 small onions, sliced

Method:

1. Mix together all the seasoning ingredients in a bowl. Sprinkle over the chicken pieces.
2. Place it in a bowl. Add scallions, hot pepper, thyme, tomatoes, garlic, thyme and onions and stir

3. Place a Dutch oven or skillet over medium heat. Add oil and allow it to heat.
4. Remove only the chicken pieces from the bowl and add a few pieces at a time and cook until brown.
5. Add the cooked chicken into another skillet. Add the other ingredients that were in the bowl along with the chicken.
6. Add ketchup and water and stir. Place the skillet over medium heat.
7. When it begins to boil, lower heat and cover with a lid. Simmer until the gravy is thickened.
8. Serve over rice or anything of your choice.

Servings: 6

Ingredients:

- 3 cups frozen spinach, thawed
- 1 finely diced small yellow onion (you will get about 1 cup)
- 2 cups aged Gouda cheese (grated)
- 3 table-spoons butter (unsalted)
- Kosher salt and freshly crushed pepper, to taste
- 1/8 tea-spoon nutmeg (freshly grated)
- 1 1/2 cups heavy cream

Method:

1. Thaw the frozen spinach and strain through a colander.
2. Wrap the drained spinach in a cheesecloth or cloth towel and squeeze out the liquid from the spinach.
3. Heat butter over medium heat in a large skillet (straight-sided one) and add the onions to the melted butter.
4. Stir-fry the onions for 8 minutes until translucent and tender. Add kosher salt and pepper. Mix well.
5. Add the grated nutmeg and heavy cream to the skillet; continue to cook for 3 minutes until the cream gets reduced by half.
6. Add the grated cheese to the creamy onion mixture and stir until the cheese melts.
7. Now, add the spinach and mix well until the flavors blend and the mixture is well-incorporated.
8. Cover the skillet and cook for 10 minutes over medium-low heat until the spinach becomes soft and tender.
9. Add more salt and pepper as desired. Mix well for one last time and transfer to a bowl.
10. Serve warm and enjoy!

Servings: 8

Ingredients:

- 2 tea-spoons ground cumin
- 1 tea-spoon ground turmeric
- 8 chicken breast halves, skinless, boneless
- Pepper to taste
- Salt to taste
- 4 table-spoons olive oil
- 2 table-spoons fresh ginger, minced
- 4 cloves garlic, minced
- 2 cans light coconut milk
- 2 tea-spoons ground cayenne pepper
- 2 tea-spoons ground coriander
- 2 onions, chopped
- 4 jalapeño peppers, chopped
- 6 tomatoes, chopped
- 2 bunches fresh parsley, chopped

Method:

1. Add cumin, turmeric, cayenne pepper, and coriander into a bowl and stir.
2. Sprinkle salt and pepper over the chicken. Rub the spice mixture over the chicken.
3. Select 'Sauté' button. Add 2 table-spoons oil. When the oil is heated, add chicken and sauté until brown. Remove chicken with a slotted spoon. Set aside.
4. Add remaining oil. When the oil is heated, add onion, ginger, jalapeño pepper and garlic. Sauté until onions are translucent.
5. Add tomatoes and cook for 3-4 minutes. Add coconut milk and chicken into the pot. Mix well.
6. Close the lid. Select 'Poultry' button.
7. When the timer goes off, let the pressure release naturally.
8. Sprinkle parsley and stir.

9. Serve hot.

Servings: 4

Ingredients

<u>For the filling:</u>

- ½ table-spoon coconut oil
- 1 clove garlic, minced
- ¼ tea-spoon dried thyme
- ¼ tea-spoon ground cumin
- 1/8 tea-spoon ground allspice
- 1/8 tea-spoon ground turmeric
- Paprika to taste
- ¼ cup onions, finely chopped
- 1 small spring onion, chopped
- ¼ cup brown lentils, rinsed
- ½ table-spoon tamari or coconut aminos
- Salt to taste
- Cayenne pepper to taste (optional)
- 1 cup water or vegetable broth

<u>For crust:</u>

- 1 cup oat flour
- 2 table-spoons potato starch
- ½ tea-spoon baking powder
- 1 tea-spoon curry powder
- 2 table-spoons tapioca flour
- ½ table-spoon ground flax seeds
- ¼ tea-spoon salt
- ¼ cup almond milk

Method:

1. Place a saucepan over medium high heat. Add oil. When the oil is heated, add onion, garlic and spring onion and sauté until onions are translucent.
2. Add thyme, spices and lentils and stir until the lentils are well coated in the mixture.
3. Pour water and stir. When it begins to boil, lower heat and cover with a lid.
4. Simmer until tender and nearly dry.
5. Add tamari, salt and cayenne pepper and stir.
6. Turn off the heat and cool for a while.
7. To make crust: Add all the dry ingredients into a bowl. Add vegan butter and cut with a pastry cutter or with your hands until crumbly in texture.
8. Add almond milk and mix using your hands and form dough.
9. Divide the dough into 4 equal portions and shape into balls.
10. Place a ball between 2 pieces of parchment paper and roll into a disc of about 4-inch diameter.
11. Place 1 table-spoon of the lentil mixture on one half of the disc. Fold the other half over it, lifting along with the parchment paper. Press with a fork to seal the edges
12. Repeat the above 3 steps with the remaining 3 balls of dough.
13. Bake in a preheated oven at 400° F for 25-30 minutes or until golden brown in color.
14. Serve hot or warm.

Servings: 10

Ingredients:

- 3 3/4 pounds thinly sliced (1/4 inch) chuck roast (10 strips)
- 1/4 cup cornstarch
- 16 strips of bacon
- 1 thinly sliced large onion
- 1 tea-spoon yellow mustard paste
- 1 tea-spoon pepper (freshly ground)
- 3 cups water, divided
- 1/2 cup vegetable oil
- 1 tea-spoon sea salt
- Sour cream, optional

Method:

1. Spread a thin layer of mustard paste on the chuck roast strips and sprinkle pepper and salt over it.
2. Put one or two strips of bacon on the meat (ensure the bacon doesn't stick out in the side). Cover the bacon with sliced onions (thin layer should do).
3. Start rolling the meat from the small end along with its contents to form a tight cylinder.
4. Pour 3 table-spoons of oil on a heavy-bottomed sauté pan and add the rolled meat cylinder on the hot oil.
5. Cook for 35 minutes until all the rouladen turns golden brown and place them in a large Dutch oven.
6. Heat 2 cups of water in a small pan and pour the hot water into the same heavy-bottomed sauté pan.
7. Scrape the drippings in the pan to form the gravy. Pour this gravy sauce over the meat in the Dutch oven.
8. Add water to cover 2/3rd of the meat and bring it to boil on a stovetop. Reduce the heat, cover and simmer on low for 1-½ hours.
9. When the meat is cooked and turns tender, transfer to a plate and cover it with foil.

10. Take a small bowl and whisk 1/4-cup water and 1/4 cup cornstarch until smooth and creamy.
11. Add 1/2 of the whisked cream to the Dutch oven (you will find the juices of the cooked meat remaining in it) and whisk again until the mixture is incorporated.
12. Turn on the heat and simmer until the mixture thickens. Add 1/4-cup sour cream before serving.
13. Transfer the rouladen pieces (one per plate) to the plate and pour the prepared gravy generously.
14. Serve with pasta, potatoes, corn or broccoli. Enjoy!

Servings: 6

Ingredients:

- 2 tea-spoons turmeric powder
- 2 tea-spoons cumin powder
- 3 tea-spoons salt
- 2 tea-spoons ground coriander
- 2-3 tea-spoons cayenne pepper
- 9 chicken fillets, boneless, skinless
- 1 large onion, chopped
- 3 table-spoons olive oil
- 3 tea-spoons ginger, minced
- 3 cloves garlic, minced
- 1 ½ cans (14 ounces each) coconut milk
- 4 small jalapeño peppers, deseeded, chopped
- 5 fresh tomatoes, deseeded
- 6 cups baby spinach

Method:

1. Select 'Sauté' button. Add 1-½ table-spoons of oil and let it heat.
2. Dry the chicken with paper towels. Mix together all the spices in a bowl. Sprinkle the spice mixture over the chicken.
3. Place chicken in the instant pot. Cook until brown. Remove chicken with a slotted spoon and set aside in a bowl. Cover with foil. Set aside for a while.
4. Add remaining oil. When the oil heats, add onion, ginger, garlic and jalapeño and sauté until translucent.
5. Add coconut milk and chicken and stir.
6. Close the lid. Select 'Poultry' button and set the timer for 15 minutes.
7. When the timer goes off, let the pressure release naturally for 3-4 minutes after which quick release excess pressure.
8. Add spinach and stir. Cover and let it sit for a while.
9. Taste and adjust the seasoning if necessary.

10. Serving option: Rice.

Servings: 6-8 Servings

Ingredients

- 1 pound saltfish (cod fish), boneless
- 2 ripe tomatoes, sliced
- 2 cloves garlic, sliced or crushed
- 8 tea-spoons vegetable oil
- 2 table-spoons ketchup
- Hot pepper to taste
- 1 onion, sliced
- 2 cans (10 ounces each) baked beans, drained
- Water, as required

Method:

1. Soak the saltfish overnight or for about 8 hours by submerging it in cold water in order to remove the excess salt. Throughout this time period, drain out the water and add fresh water a few times.
2. Remove the scales from the saltfish.
3. Add some cold water to a pan and bring it to a boil over high heat. Once it starts boiling, bring the heat down to medium low and add in the saltfish. Allow it to simmer gently for about 25 minutes or until the fish is tender.
4. When done, remove the fish and shred into smaller pieces.
5. Place a Dutch oven or a deep skillet over medium low heat. Add oil. When the oil is heated, add onion, tomato, garlic and hot pepper and stir-fry until onions are soft.
6. Add saltfish and stir. Cook for a minute.
7. Add rest of the ingredients and stir.
8. Lower heat and cover with a lid. Simmer for 2-3 minutes. Turn off the heat.
9. It can be served right away or cooled for a few minutes and served later.

Servings: 8

Ingredients:

- 3 eggs
- 1 sliced onion
- 1 1/2 cups all-purpose flour
- 1 1/2 cups Emmentaler cheese (shredded)
- 3/8 cup 2 percent milk
- 3/4 tea-spoon nutmeg (ground)
- 3 table-spoons butter
- 3/4 tea-spoon salt
- 1/8 tea-spoon pepper

Method:

1. Sift the nutmeg, flour, pepper and salt together in a small bowl.
2. Take another medium bowl and beat the eggs well. Add the milk and flour mixture alternately to the eggs. Beat them until smooth and let it stand for 30 minutes.
3. Boil water and 1/2-tea-spoon salt in a large pot. Press the prepared batter into the water through a Spaetzle press or potato ricer. Let it cook.
4. Remove the Spaetzle with a slotted spoon when it floats on top of the water to a bowl. Mix 1 cup of cheese to the cooked Spaetzle.
5. Take a large skillet and melt the butter over medium-high heat. Add the onion and fry till it turns golden brown.
6. Add the cheese-mixed Spaetzle to the skillet and mix well. You can add the remaining cheese (if any) and stir well until it blends well.
7. Transfer to a plate and serve immediately.

Servings: 3

Ingredients:

- 2 tea-spoons extra-virgin olive oil
- ¼ tea-spoon ground cumin
- ¼ tea-spoon ground turmeric
- ¼ tea-spoon cayenne pepper
- ¼ tea-spoon ground coriander
- 3 chicken breasts, skinless, boneless
- 3 table-spoons fresh ginger, thinly sliced
- 1 table-spoon fresh lemon juice
- 1 cup jarred or boxed unsalted tomatoes, divided
- ½ cup light coconut milk
- 2 cloves garlic, minced, divided
- 1 small jalapeño pepper, deseeded, sliced
- A handful fresh cilantro, chopped + extra to garnish
- 1 small onion, chopped
- ¼ cup low sodium chicken broth
- 2 table-spoons shredded coconut, unsweetened, toasted

Method:

1. Add all the spices, oil, and half the garlic in a bowl. Mix well and add chicken. Turn the chicken in the mixture to coat well.
2. Add cilantro, jalapeño pepper, ginger and remaining half garlic into a food processor and pulse until very tiny pieces are formed. Pour lemon juice and blend again until well combined.
3. Select 'Sauté' button. Add oil. When the oil is heated, add chicken and sauté until brown on all the sides. Remove and set aside on a plate.
4. Add onions and sauté until light brown. Add the cilantro mixture and cook for a couple of minutes. Stir frequently.
5. Press 'Cancel' button.

6. Transfer all the mixture that is in the instant pot into a blender. Also add broth and ½ cup tomatoes and blend for 45-50 seconds or until smooth. Pour into the instant pot.
7. Add remaining tomatoes and stir until well combined. Add chicken and stir.
8. Close the lid. Select 'Poultry' button and set the timer for 10 minutes.
9. When the timer goes off, quick release excess pressure. Pour milk and stir.
10. Select 'Sauté' button and press 'Adjust' button twice. Simmer until the sauce is thickened as per your desire.
11. Serve with shredded coconut and cilantro garnished on top.

Servings: 6 Servings

Ingredients

- 3 pounds smoked ham leg bone in
- 5-6 cloves
- 1-2 table-spoons smoky jerk marinade

For glaze:

- 2 table-spoons honey
- ½ tea-spoon brown sugar
- ½ tea-spoon ginger powder
- ½ cup coca –cola
- 1 tea-spoon cornstarch mixed in water
- Salt to taste

Method:

1. Discard all the packaging material and place ham in a roasting pan. Pour 2-3 cups water all around the ham.
2. Wrap tightly with ham and place it in the oven.
3. Let it cook in a preheated oven at 350° F. The time for cooking is approximately 20-25 minutes per pound of meat.
4. Discard skin and remove excess fat. Score the meat all over with a sharp knife. The cuts should go through the fat as well as a little in the meat.
5. Rub jerk marinade all over. Insert the cloves in the slits.
6. Place it back in the oven for 15 minutes.
7. Meanwhile, place a saucepan with all the glaze ingredients over low heat. Stir until well combined.
8. Remove meat from the oven and brush glaze all over it.
9. Roast for another 15 minutes.
10. Slice and serve.

Servings: 8

Ingredients:

- 4 pounds chuck roast (trim the excess fat and pat dry)
- 2 chopped onions,
- 2 chopped celery ribs
- 4 chopped carrots
- 4 minced garlic cloves
- 1 cup dry red wine
- 1 cup gingersnap cookies (finely crushed)
- 3 table-spoons vegetable oil
- 1/2 tea-spoon cloves (ground)
- 1/2 cup brown sugar
- 1/2 cup red wine vinegar
- 1 tea-spoon salt
- 2 bay leaves
- 1/2 cup water
- 1 tea-spoon pepper

Method:

1. Rub the salt and pepper over the roast and keep it aside.
2. Heat oil in a pressure cooker and cook the chuck roast until all the sides turn brown (use the *brown* function in the cooker or roast the meat without the lid if it is an old-fashioned cooker).
3. Take a small bowl and mix the wine, water, vinegar, bay leaves, cloves, salt and sugar until combined well.
4. Place the gingersnaps and chopped vegetables around the browned roast; pour the vinegar mixture over the entire contents.
5. Close the cooker, raise the pressure to high and let it cook for 55 minutes.
6. Let the pressure release naturally after the meat is done (don't manually release the pressure).

7. Open the lid when the pressure drops and transfer the meat (only the roast not the vegetables) to a plate. Remove the bay leaves and cover it with a foil.
8. Pour the cooked vegetables and sauce in a high-speed blender and blend until smooth.
9. Remove the foil of the meat and serve with the blended sauce.

Servings: 6

Ingredients:

- 6 table-spoons vinegar
- 3 tea-spoons paprika
- 1 ½ table-spoons vegetable oil
- 7-8 tomatoes, chopped
- 1 tea-spoon salt
- 1 ½ table-spoons garlic, chopped
- 12 chicken thighs, skin-on, trimmed
- 5 large onions, chopped
- 3 bay leaves
- 3-4 table-spoons water or more if required

Method:

1. Add vinegar, paprika and garlic into a large bowl and stir.
2. Add chicken and coat it well on all the sides. Cover and place in the refrigerator for 1-1½ hours.
3. Select 'Sauté' button. Add oil. When the oil is heated, add onions and fry till golden brown.
4. Discard the marinating mixture of the chicken and add chicken into the instant pot. Cook until brown.
5. Add rest of the ingredients and stir. Press 'Cancel' button.
6. Close the lid. Select 'Poultry' button and set the timer for 10 minutes.
7. When the timer goes off, quick release excess pressure.

Servings: 4 Servings

Ingredients:

- 2 pounds package cut chicken wings
- 1 tea-spoon smoky paprika
- Oil, as required, to fry
- 1 table-spoon brown sugar
- ½ cup flour
- 4 table-spoons BBQ sauce or more to taste
- ¼ tea-spoon salt or to taste
- Pepper to taste

Method:

1. Line 1- 3 baking sheets with parchment paper.
2. Trim the chicken of excess fat. Cut off the tips of each wing. Trim the skin. Dry with paper towels.
3. Add pepper, salt and paprika into a bowl and mix well. Sprinkle this mixture over the wings.
4. Coat the wings in flour.
5. Place a shallow pan over medium heat. Add oil and let it heat. It should be well heated but not smoking.
6. Add wings in batches and fry until crisp.
7. Remove with a slotted spoon and place on a plate lined with paper towels.
8. Place wings in a bowl. Pour BBQ sauce over it. Toss well and serve right away.

Servings: 5

Ingredients:

- 2 Eggs
- 7 medium starchy potatoes (grated)
- 1/3 cups Plain flour
- 1 grated brown onion
- 1 table-spoon butter
- 1 table-spoon olive oil
- 1/2 tea-spoon Salt

Method:

1. Take a large bowl and mix the grated onions and potatoes.
2. Crack 2 eggs and lightly beat them.
3. Add the beaten eggs, 1/3 cup flour and salt to the bowl of grated onions and potatoes.
4. Mix together well until combined.
5. Heat the olive oil and butter in a frying pan.
6. Scoop out 1/4 cup of the mixture and flatten them a little bit.
7. Place this in the hot oil and fry for 8 minutes until both the side turn golden.
8. Drain on paper towels and serve with sauce. Enjoy!

Servings: 6

Ingredients:

- 4 ½ table-spoons olive oil, divided
- 4 ½ cups mushrooms, sliced
- 3 chicken breasts, skinless, boneless, thinly sliced
- 1 ½ cans (14.5 ounces each) canned stewed tomatoes, blended
- 2 onions, thinly sliced
- 3 cloves garlic, crushed
- Salt to taste
- Pepper to taste
- 1 ½ cans table cream (7.6 ounces)

Method:

1. Select 'Sauté' button. Add oil. When the oil is heated, add onions and fry till onions are translucent.
2. Add chicken and cook for 3-4 minutes.
3. Stir in the mushrooms and garlic and cook for a couple of minutes. Add salt, pepper, and tomatoes and stir. Press 'Cancel' button.
4. Close the lid. Select 'Poultry' button and set the timer for 15 minutes.
5. When the timer goes off, quick release excess pressure.
6. Serve with hot cooked rice, preferably white rice and potato sticks.

Servings: 2

Ingredients

- 1 table-spoon unsalted butter
- 2 cloves garlic, minced
- 1 shallot, minced
- ½ cup Myer's dark rum
- 1 table-spoon ancho puree
- Salt to taste
- Freshly ground pepper to taste
- 1 ½ cups chicken stock
- 1 table-spoon molasses
- 2 filet mignon steaks (8 ounces each)

Method:

1. Place a saucepan over medium high heat. Add butter. When butter melts, add garlic and shallots and sauté until translucent.
2. Add rum and boil until it reduces to 4-5 table-spoons.
3. Stir in the stock. When it begins to boil, lower heat and continue simmering until it reduces to about a cup.
4. Meanwhile, preheat a grill. Sprinkle salt and pepper over the steaks and place on the grill.
5. Grill until the way you like it cooked.
6. Pour the cooked sauce over the steak and serve.

Servings: 6

Ingredients:

- 6 chicken breasts (boneless and skinless)
- 1 chopped onion
- 1 1/2 cups chicken stock
- 4 minced garlic cloves
- 1/3 cup flour
- 2 tea-spoons paprika
- 1 1/2 cups sour cream
- 3 table-spoons tomato paste
- 2 table-spoons peanut oil
- 1 table-spoon cornstarch
- 1 table-spoon butter
- 1 tea-spoon salt
- 1 tea-spoon smoked paprika
- 1/8 tea-spoon white pepper

Method:

1. Take a shallow plate and mix the flour, pepper, 2 tea-spoons paprika and salt until combined well. Dip the chicken breasts into the mixture and coat well on both sides.
2. Heat the butter and peanut oil in a heavy-bottomed skillet over medium heat. Add the coated chicken and cook for 5 minutes until both the sides turn brown.
3. Once all the chicken breasts are done, transfer to a plate and set aside.
4. Add the garlic and onion to the same skillet and stir-fry until they turn tender and crisp.
5. Add the tomato paste and the chicken stock into the skillet. Stir the contents until they combine well. Bring it to boil.
6. Place the cooked chicken back to the skillet and cover it with a lid. Lower the heat and simmer for 10 minutes.
7. Take another small bowl and mix the cornstarch, sour cream and the smoked paprika until they combine well.

8. Add this mixture into the skillet when the chicken is cooked thoroughly and heat through it (do not boil!)
9. Serve with hot cooked rice or mashed potatoes.

Servings: 6

Ingredients:

- 1 large whole chicken, cut into parts
- 4-5 large tomatoes, chopped
- 6 cloves garlic, grated
- 1 ¼ cups coconut milk
- ½ table-spoon coriander
- 2 table-spoons turmeric
- A pinch cayenne pepper
- 1 large onion, chopped
- 1 inch fresh ginger, peeled, grated
- 1 ½ table-spoons tomato puree
- 1 ½ cans tinned tomatoes
- 1 ½ table-spoons basil
- 3 table-spoons cumin
- Salt to taste
- Pepper to taste

Method:

1. Add all the ingredients except coconut milk into the instant pot and stir.
2. Close the lid. Select 'Poultry' button and set the timer for 12 minutes.
3. When the clock goes off, let the pressure release naturally.
4. Add coconut milk and mix well.
5. Serve in bowls.

Servings: 6

Ingredients:

- 1 container chicken broth
- 1/4 cup finely chopped onions
- 2 beaten eggs
- 1/2 cup chopped celery
- 4 cups bread cubes
- 1/2 tea-spoon poultry seasoning
- 1/3 cup butter
- 1/2 tea-spoon sage
- 1/8 tea-spoon black pepper
- 1/2 tea-spoon salt

Method:

1. Preheat the oven to 325 F. Grease the baking dish with butter (be generous while greasing)
2. Warmth butter in a fry pan over medium heat. Add onion and celery to the pan, sauté until the mixture softens.
3. Transfer the cooked onion-celery mixture into a large bowl. Add the bread cubes, poultry seasoning, sage, pepper and salt. Mix well until combined.
4. Add the broth to the mixture and stir until all the contents are moistened well. Check for taste and add salt accordingly.
5. Beat the eggs in a separate bowl and add it to the broth mixture. Stir until all the contents blend well.
6. Pour the batter into the lubricated baking bowl. Pack it loosely and cover the dish with the foil tightly.
7. Bake for 45 minutes and then remove the foil.
8. Bake again for another 10 minutes until browned.
9. Serve hot.

Servings: 8

Ingredients:

- 6 table-spoons oil
- 2 table-spoons annatto seed paste
- 12 cloves garlic, smashed
- ½ cup fresh cilantro, chopped
- 2 tomatoes, quartered
- 2 bay leaves
- 2/3 cup green olives, sliced
- 2 cups fresh or frozen corn
- 6 bone-in split chicken breasts with skin
- Salt to taste
- 1 red pepper, cut into thin strips
- 2 white onions, chopped
- 8 cups water, divided
- Cooked rice to serve
- 4 table-spoons Media Crema table cream

Method:

1. Add oil into the instant pot. Swirl the pot to spread oil.
2. Place chicken with its skin side facing down.
3. Add garlic, cilantro, red pepper and tomato into a blender and blend until smooth. Add half the water and blend again. Pour into the instant pot over the chicken.
4. Pour remaining water over the chicken.
5. Close the lid. Select 'Poultry' button. Once the clock goes off, let the pressure release naturally.
6. Drain most of the cooked liquid but retain some.
7. Remove chicken from the pot and place on your cutting board. When cool enough to handle, shred the chicken and add it back into the pot.
8. Add the retained liquid, corn, olives and cream and stir.
9. Serve over rice.

Servings: 8 pies

Ingredients:

- 1 tea-spoon fresh thyme leaves, chopped
- 1 clove garlic, chopped
- 1 small green bell pepper, deseeded, chopped
- 1 tea-spoon Jamaican curry powder
- 1 table-spoon vegetable oil
- 1 package (17.3 ounces) puff pastry
- Barbecue sauce or chutney or ranch dressing to serve
- 3 scallions, chopped
- 1 small scotch bonnet chili or habanero, deseeded, chopped
- 4 ounces ground beef
- 1/8 tea-spoon ground allspice
- Freshly ground pepper to taste
- Salt to taste
- 1 small egg, beaten with a table-spoon water

Method:

1. Add thyme, garlic, bell pepper and scallions into the food processor bowl and pulse until finely chopped.
2. Place a nonstick skillet over medium heat. Add beef and cook until light brown.
3. Add the finely chopped vegetables, allspice and curry powder and cook until beef is brown. Turn off the heat.
4. Add oil, salt and pepper and stir. Taste and adjust the seasoning if necessary. Cool completely.
5. Dust your countertop with a little flour. Place the puff pastry sheets and roll until it is 1/8 inch thick.
6. Use an oval shaped cutter and cut out 4 ovals from each of the pastry sheets. Set aside the scraps.
7. Place 1 table-spoon of the beef mixture on the center of 4 of the ovals. Brush egg on the edges. Cover with the remaining 4 ovals. Seal the edges with a fork.
8. Place the ovals on a baking sheet lined with baking paper.

9. Now cut 8 strips of 2 x 1/8 inch from the dough scrap and 24 strips of 1 x 1/8 inch strip.
10. Place the long strips along the length of the patties and the short strips crosswise in such a manner that it resembles a football.
11. Brush with egg.
12. Bake in a preheated oven at 350° F for 35-45 minutes or until golden brown. When done, let it sit for 10 minutes.
13. Serve meat pie footballs with ranch dressing or barbecue sauce as a dip.

Servings: 6

Ingredients:

- 3 cups Emmentaler cheese (shredded)
- 3 cups (12 ounces) dry Spätzle (cooked)
- 2 sliced small onions
- 2 table-spoon olive oil
- Salt and pepper to taste

Method:

1. Preheat the oven to 325 F.
2. Warmth the olive oil in a skillet over average heat. Add the onions and sauté for 10 minutes until it becomes translucent and brown.
3. Grease the casserole dish and layer with 1/2 Spätzle. Season with pepper and salt.
4. Prepare the next layer by sprinkling 1/2 of the shredded cheese and again another ½ layer Spätzle and end it with 1/2 layer of cheese.
5. Top the casserole with sautéed onions and back for 35 minutes uncovered.
6. You can transfer to a plate once the casserole becomes bubbly and turns brown on the top.
7. Serve warm and enjoy!

Servings: 2-3

Ingredients:

- 1.5 pounds beef chuck, cut into 1-inch chops.
- 3 large tomatoes, cut into wedges
- 2 cloves garlic, minced
- 2 cans (13 ½ ounces each) coconut milk, unsweetened
- ½ table-spoon red pepper flakes
- Pepper to taste
- Salt to taste
- A handful fresh cilantro, chopped, to garnish
- 2 table-spoons olive oil
- 1 medium yellow onion, chopped
- 1 tea-spoon fresh ginger, grated
- ½ table-spoon dried oregano
- 9-10 ounces canned black beans, drained, rinsed

Method:

1. Select 'Sauté' button. Add beef and cook until brown.
2. Add onion, ginger, tomato and garlic and sauté for a couple of minutes.
3. Add rest of the ingredients and stir. Press 'Cancel' button.
4. Close the lid. Select 'Meat / Stew' button. Set the timer for 50 minutes.
5. Once the clock goes off, let the pressure release naturally.
6. Add cilantro and stir.
7. Serve hot.

Servings: 8-10

Ingredients:

<u>For coconut rice:</u>

- 2 table-spoons vegetable oil
- 2 ½ cups coconut milk
- ½ cup fresh cilantro, chopped
- 4 cups basmati rice, rinsed, drained
- 2 tea-spoons kosher salt
- 4 scallions, thinly sliced

<u>For jerk sauce:</u>

- 6 table-spoons vegetable oil
- 2 inches piece fresh ginger, peeled, minced
- 8 cloves garlic, minced
- 2 scotch bonnet peppers, halved
- 2 fresh bay leaves
- 2 bunches scallions, chopped, set aside a little for garnishing
- 1 tea-spoon ground cinnamon
- 4 tea-spoons ground allspice
- 1 tea-spoon nutmeg, grated
- Kosher salt to taste
- 1 cup chicken stock
- 6 table-spoons soy sauce
- Juice of 4 limes
- Zest of 2 limes, grated
- ¼ cup fresh thyme, chopped
- ½ cup fresh cilantro, chopped
- 1 cup dark brown sugar

<u>For lobster:</u>

- 2 sticks unsalted butter, at room temperature
- 8 lobster tails (10-12 ounces each), halved lengthwise

Method:

1. To make coconut rice: Place a large saucepan (that has a tight fitting lid) over medium heat.
2. Add oil. When the oil is heated, add rice and sauté for a few minutes until opaque.
3. Add coconut milk, 3 cups water, salt and stir. When it begins to boil, simmer until the water is almost the same as the rice.
4. Cover with a tight fitting lid and lower heat to low heat. Let the rice cook for 15 minutes.
5. Stir and cover again. Remove from heat. Using a fork, fluff the rice. Stir in scallions and cilantro.
6. To make jerk sauce: Place a saucepan over medium high heat. Add oil. When the oil is heated, add ginger, garlic, and scallions and scotch bonnet chili and sauté until fragrant.
7. Add all the spices, salt and fresh bay leaf. Sauté for a few seconds until fragrant.
8. Add brown sugar, thyme, stock, soy sauce and zest. Let it cook for 7-8 minutes.
9. Add lime juice and half the cilantro.
10. Set aside half the sauce for dipping.
11. To make lobster: Set a grill to preheat to medium high heat. Coat a little of the remaining sauce on the flesh side of the lobster. Place lobster on the grill, with the flesh side facing down.
12. Grill until golden brown. It should take around 5 minutes. Turn sides and baste again with remaining sauce. Cook until the flesh begins to come away from the shells.
13. Spread coconut rice on a serving platter. Place lobster tails over the rice.
14. Brush lobster tails with a little butter. Drizzle remaining jerk sauce all over the rice and sprinkle cilantro and scallion greens.

Servings: 6

Ingredients:

- 1 pound quartered mushrooms (fresh)
- 12 ounces spaghetti
- 4 ounces cubed mozzarella
- 3 chopped green onions
- 2 precooked smoked sausage (cubed)
- 1 minced garlic clove
- 24 ounces pasta sauce (1 can)
- 5 table-spoons olive oil
- Salt, pepper to taste

Method:

1. Preheat oven to 400 F.
2. Cook the spaghetti in a pot as per the package instructions until it is firm to bite. Drain and rinse with cold water.
3. Transfer the spaghetti back to the pot and add 3 table-spoons of olive oil. Mix well and set aside.
4. Heat the remaining olive oil in a frying pan and add the mushrooms. Stir-fry until it browns.
5. Add the sausage to the pan and stir-fry until it turns brown. Add the garlic and onion; continue to stir-fry until tender and brown. Cook for few minutes and remove from heat.
6. Take a casserole dish and put 1/3 of pasta sauce to the bottom. Divide the spaghetti into 7 portions and form noodle nests.
7. Place a portion on a sauce and twirl it around with a fork from the nest with a depression in the center. Slide the nest into the casserole dish.
8. Repeat step 7 with the remaining spaghetti.
9. Pour the mushroom mixture into the center of the 7 nests and pour the remaining pasta sauce around the nests.
10. Sprinkle the mozzarella over the top and bake uncovered for 35 minutes until it turns bubbly.

11. Transfer to plate and serve hot.

Servings: 10

Ingredients:

- 1 pound beef chuck, cut into 2 inch cubes
- 2 table-spoons red wine vinegar
- ½ table-spoon coarse spicy mustard
- 2 small onion, chop 1 and slice 1
- 1 medium tomato, deseeded, chopped
- 1 small green bell pepper, cut into strips
- 2 table-spoons vegetable oil
- ½ table-spoon soy sauce
- ½ tea-spoon Worcestershire sauce
- 1 clove garlic, minced
- 1 table-spoon tomato paste
- ½ tea-spoon dried oregano
- 1 table-spoon cachaca or rum or water
- Hot sauce to taste (optional)
- 1 green onion, thinly sliced
- 2 table-spoons vegetable oil
- ½ table-spoon soy sauce
- ½ tea-spoon Worcestershire sauce
- ½ table-spoon beef bouillon paste or ½ -1 cup beef stock
- ½ table-spoon corn starch
- ½ table-spoon capers
- 10 sandwich rolls to serve

Method:

1. Add vegetable oil, soy sauce, vinegar and mustard in a small glass bowl. Whisk well.
2. Add beef and stir until well combined. Cover the bowl with plastic wrap loosely. Place in the refrigerator for 7-8.
3. Select 'Sauté' button and let the instant pot heat.
4. Remove beef with a slotted spoon and place in the instant pot. Keep aside the marinade.

5. Cook until beef is brown. Remove with a spoon and set aside on a plate.
6. Add chopped onions into the instant pot. Sauté until translucent. Add garlic and sauté until fragrant.
7. Add tomatoes and sauté for a couple of minutes. Add sliced onions, tomato paste, oregano and green pepper and sauté for a couple of minutes.
8. Add beef back into the pot. Add beef bouillon and enough water to cover (water need not be added if you are using beef stock). Press 'Cancel' button.
9. Close the lid. Select 'Slow cook' button and set the timer for 2 hours or until beef is cooked through.
10. Remove beef with a slotted spoon and place on your cutting board. Shred with a pair of forks. Add it back into the pot.
11. Add cachaca, cornstarch and hot sauce into a bowl and whisk well.
12. Add into the instant pot.
13. Select 'Sauté' button and stir constantly until the mixture thickens.
14. Add capers and green onions and mix well.
15. Place in between sandwich rolls and serve.

Servings: 6 Servings

Ingredients:

- 3 pounds leg of lamb, boneless, butterflied, halved along the length
- 2 table-spoons dried thyme
- Kosher salt to taste
- ½ table-spoon sherry vinegar
- 1 scallion, sliced
- 1 small red bell pepper, deseeded, chopped
- ¼ cup extra virgin olive oil
- 1 tea-spoon ground allspice
- ½ table-spoon dark brown sugar
- ½ tea-spoon fresh ginger, peeled, grated
- ½ cup ripe papaya pieces, peeled, deseeded
- 1 small habanero pepper, deseed if desired, minced

Method:

1. Set a grill to preheat to medium high heat.
2. Brush half the oil over the lamb. Rub ½ table-spoon thyme on each side of the lamb leg pieces. Also rub ¼ tea-spoon allspice and salt liberally on each side of the lamb pieces.
3. Place lamb with the fat side down on the grill. Cook until brown. Flip sides and cook the other side until brown or the internal temperature of meat in the thickest part shows 125 - 135 ° F according to the way you like it cooked.
4. When done, place lamb on your chopping board. Cover lamb with foil, loosely. Let it sit for 10 minutes. Slice the lamb and place on individual serving plates.
5. Meanwhile, add remaining oil, vinegar, brown sugar, ginger and ¼ tea-spoon salt into a bowl. Stir until sugar dissolves completely.
6. Stir in scallions, bell pepper, papaya and habanero pepper. Toss well.

7. Sprinkle some salt over the lamb and serve with papaya
   salsa.

52

Servings: 6

Ingredients:

- 2 pounds fresh asparagus (washed and dried)
- 1/4 cup Parmesan cheese (ground)
- 1/2 cup bread crumbs (seasoned)
- 1 tea-spoon freshly ground pepper
- 1/2 cup olive oil

Method:

1. Preheat oven to 400 F.
2. Pour 1/4 cup olive oil onto a cookie sheet (with rim).
3. Snap the bottom end of the dried asparagus and peel the stem if required.
4. Lay them neatly onto the cookie sheet.
5. Drizzle the oil over them all and gently turn the spring vegetable until they are completely coated with oil.
6. Sprinkle the breadcrumbs over them and then the ground Parmesan cheese.
7. Season with the freshly ground pepper and bake for 20 minutes until they turn crispy and fragrant.
8. Transfer to a plate and serve warm with any creamy dip.

Servings: 3

Ingredients:

- 1 tea-spoon canola oil
- ½ table-spoon garlic, peeled, minced
- ½ table-spoon chili powder
- ¼ tea-spoon ground cumin
- 2/3 cup unsalted chicken stock, divided
- 7.5 ounces canned pinto beans, rinsed, drained
- 7.5 ounces canned black beans, rinsed, drained
- ¼ cup fresh cilantro, chopped
- 6 tea-spoons sour cream
- 4 ounces sweet turkey Italian sausage, discard casing
- ¼ tea-spoon dried oregano
- 1 bay leaf
- 1 poblano chili, deseeded, finely chopped
- 1 can (14 ounces) diced tomatoes, with its liquid
- 1 table-spoon all-purpose flour
- Freshly ground pepper to taste
- Radish slices to serve (optional)

Method:

1. Place an oven over medium high heat. Add oil. When the oil is heated, add garlic and onion and cook until brown.
2. Add sausage, chili powder, cumin, oregano, bay leaf and poblano pepper and mix well. Break meat simultaneously as it cooks. Cook until brown.
3. Add ½ cup stock, both the beans and tomatoes.
4. When it begins to boil, lower the heat and simmer until it is slightly thick.
5. Add remaining stock into a bowl. Add flour and mix well. Pour into the pot. Stir constantly until thick.

6. Turn off the heat. Add cilantro and pepper powder. Remove the bay leaf.
7. Ladle into bowls. Drizzle 3 tea-spoons sour cream in each bowl. Place radish slices if desired and serve.

Servings: 4

Ingredients:

- 4 ounces fresh or frozen yuca (cassava), thawed, peeled, cut into ½ inch cubes
- 1 pound large shrimp, peeled, deveined
- ¼ tea-spoon salt, divided
- 1 table-spoon olive oil
- ½ cup red bell pepper, cut into slices
- ¼ cup light coconut milk
- A handful fresh cilantro, chopped
- 2 cloves garlic, peeled
- 1 table-spoon fresh lime juice
- 1 tea-spoon annatto seeds
- 1 medium onion, sliced (about a cup of onions)
- 1 ½ cups tomato, peeled, deseeded, chopped
- ½ table-spoon habanero pepper or Scotch bonnet pepper
- Lime wedges to serve
- Salt to taste

Method:

1. Place yuca in the instant pot. Pour enough water to cover it.
2. Close the lid. Select 'Manual' and set the timer for 15 minutes.
3. Once the clock goes off, let the pressure release naturally.
4. Retain about ½ cup of the cooked liquid and discard the rest. Transfer yuca into a bowl. Add 2-3 table-spoons of the retained liquid. Using a potato masher, mash the yuca until smooth. Remove any hard fibers.
5. Add garlic, shrimp, a large pinch salt into a bowl and stir. Cover and set aside for 3 minutes.
6. Select 'Sauté' button. Add oil. When the oil is heated, add annatto seeds and cook. In a few minutes the oil will turn deep orange. Stir frequently. Press 'Cancel' button. Strain the oil into a bowl.

7. Add the annatto seeds into the instant pot. Select 'Sauté' button. Add onions and bell pepper and cook until slightly soft.
8. Stir in the tomatoes and cook until the tomatoes are broken down. Stir once in a while. Mash the mixture with a potato masher.
9. Add shrimp along with habanero pepper and coconut milk. Mix well. Add mashed yucca, salt to taste and cilantro.
10. Press 'Adjust' button twice. Simmer until shrimp is cooked.
11. Serve in bowls. Sprinkle some more cilantro on top and place a lime wedge and serve.

Servings: 2

Ingredients:

- 1 tea-spoon olive oil
- 6 table-spoons chopped poblano pepper, deseeded
- 2 cups unsalted chicken stock
- 1 corn tortilla, chopped
- ¼ tea-spoon garlic powder
- ¼ tea-spoon ground coriander
- ¼ tea-spoon ground cumin
- ½ cup onion, chopped
- ½ ounce Spanish chorizo, finely chopped
- 6 ounces 93% lean ground turkey
- 7.2 ounces canned diced tomatoes, drained
- Salt to taste
- 1 small egg
- 6 table-spoons frozen corn kernels
- Cooking spray
- A handful fresh cilantro, chopped

Method:

1. Place a saucepan over medium high heat. Add oil. When the oil is heated, stir in the onion, chorizo and poblano and cook for 2 minutes.
2. Stir in the tomatoes and stock. When it begins to boil, lower the heat and add tortillas. Let it simmer.
3. Meanwhile, add ground turkey, all the spices and egg into a bowl and mix well.
4. Divide the mixture into 6 equal portions and shape into balls.
5. Place a nonstick skillet over medium heat. Spray with cooking spray. Place the meatballs in the pan. Cook until brown on all the sides.

6. Drop the meatballs into the simmering soup. Add salt and corn. Cook for 5 more minutes.
7. Ladle into soup bowls. Sprinkle cilantro on top and serve.

Servings: 6 Servings

Ingredients:

<u>For Jamaican curry powder:</u>

- 1 ½ table-spoons cumin seeds
- 1 ½ table-spoons fenugreek seeds
- 1 ½ table-spoons black peppercorns
- 2 tea-spoons whole allspice
- 1 ½ table-spoons mustard seeds
- 1 ½ table-spoons anise seeds
- 1 ½ table-spoons coriander seeds
- 1 ½ table-spoons turmeric powder

<u>For chicken curry:</u>

- 4 ½ table-spoons vegetable oil
- Coarse salt to taste
- Freshly ground pepper to taste
- 6 cloves garlic, minced
- 1 medium scotch bonnet pepper, minced
- 3 table-spoons fresh thyme, chopped
- 3 cups coconut milk
- 6 chicken legs, skinless, split
- 3 medium onions, thinly sliced
- 1 ½ table-spoon ginger, minced
- 6 table-spoons Jamaican curry powder or use as per your taste
- 4 ½ cups chicken stock
- Juice of a lime

Method:

1. To make Jamaican curry powder: Add cumin, fenugreek, mustard, coriander seeds, black peppercorns and allspice into a skillet.

2. Place the skillet over medium heat. Roast until a sweet aroma is in the air. Turn off the heat. Let it cool completely.
3. Transfer into a spice grinder and grind until fine. Add into a bowl. Add turmeric powder and stir well.
4. To make chicken curry: Sprinkle salt and pepper over the chicken.
5. Place a Dutch oven over high heat. Add oil. When the oil is heated, add chicken and cook until brown. Cook in batches if required. Remove the chicken with a slotted spoon and place on a plate lined with paper towels.
6. Place the pot back over heat. Stir in the onions, chili pepper, garlic and ginger. Sauté for a few minutes until onions are translucent.
7. Stir in thyme and curry powder and sauté for a few seconds until fragrant.
8. Add lime juice and stir. Add the chicken back into the pot. Pour stock and coconut milk.
9. When it begins to boil, lower heat and cover partially. Simmer until the chicken is well cooked and is falling off the bone. It may take 1-1½ hours. Remove any fat that may be floating on top.

Servings: 2-3

Ingredients:

- 1 onion, chopped
- 2 cloves garlic, chopped
- 1 ½ table-spoons oil
- ¼ cup natural cashew butter
- Pepper to taste
- Salt to taste
- 1 cup coconut milk
- ¼ cup dried shrimp
- 1 jalapeño pepper, chopped
- ¾ cup stock or water
- ½ cup breadcrumbs
- ½ pound shrimp, peeled, deveined
- 2 table-spoons dende oil (optional)

Method:

1. Add onion, garlic, dried shrimp and chili into a blender and blend until smooth. Add 1-2 table-spoons water if required while blending.
2. Select 'Sauté' button. Add oil. When the oil is heated, add the ground shrimp mixture and cook for 5-6 minutes.
3. Add stock and peanut butter and mix well.
4. Add shrimp and stir.
5. Close the lid. Select 'Manual' button and set the timer for 2 minutes.
6. When the timer goes off, quick release excess pressure.
7. Stir and serve.

Servings: 4

Ingredients:

- ½ pound tomatillos, remove stem and husks
- 1 cup onions, chopped
- 2 cloves garlic, sliced
- 1 can white hominy (15 ounces), drained
- ¼ cup cilantro, chopped
- 4 lime wedges
- 1 ½ pounds chicken breasts, halved, skinned
- 3 cups brown chicken stock
- 1 jalapeño pepper, seeded, quartered
- ½ tea-spoon salt or to taste
- 2 table-spoons reduced fat sour cream

Method:

1. Place a pot of water over average heat. When it begins to boil, add whole tomatillos and cook until tender.
2. Drain and blend the tomatillos until smooth.
3. Place the pot back on heat. Add stock, onions, chicken breasts, garlic, hominy and pepper.
4. When it begins to boil, lower heat and simmer until the chicken is cooked. Remove chicken with a slotted spoon and place on your cutting board. Shred chicken with a pair of forks and discard the bones. Add it back in the pot.
5. Add blended tomatillos and salt. Simmer for 6-7 minutes.
6. Ladle into soup bowls. Garnish with cilantro, sour cream, and lime wedges. Serve hot.

Pork Stew

Servings: 2-3

Ingredients:

- 12 ounces of pork – cut it into 1" sized pieces
- 4 table-spoons of ketchup
- 1 table-spoon of soy sauce
- 4 table-spoons of water
- ½ of 1 19 ounce can of pineapple tidbits – drained (preserve the syrup or juice)
- Pepper to taste
- ½ of sweet green pepper, chopped
- 1 table-spoon of vinegar
- ½ of a medium sized onion, chopped
- ½ table-spoon of oil
- 1 table-spoon of brown sugar
- ½ tea-spoon of salt
- 1 table-spoon of cornstarch

Method:

1. In a medium-sized saucepan, heat some oil over medium heat and add in the onions and pork.
2. Brown them gently; this will take a few minutes to achieve.
3. Take the cornstarch, sugar, and salt in a mixing bowl and combine. Slowly add in the soy sauce, vinegar, water, ketchup, and the juice or syrup preserved from the pineapple.
4. Add the mixture to the pork and stir. Allow it to cook on a low heat and keep stirring until it is clear and thick in consistency.
5. Cover the saucepan and allow it to simmer for around 1 hour.
6. Once done, add in the green pepper and pineapple tidbits then let it cook for another 7 minutes.
7. Serve with steaming hot rice.

Servings:

Ingredients:

- Pork linguica sausages, cut into small pieces
- 2 cloves garlic, minced
- 3 cups water
- ½ cup cornmeal
- 3-4 collard leaves, cut into strips
- 1 medium onion, sliced
- 1 tea-spoon hot pepper flakes
- 1 meat bouillon cubes
- 1 tea-spoon salt

For mashed plantain:

- 2 ripe plantains
- 2 table-spoons butter, milk or half and half
- ¼ cup coconut milk
- ¼ cup Parmesan cheese, grated

Method:

1. Select 'Sauté' button. Add sausages and sauté until well cooked.
2. Stir in the onion and sauté until translucent. Stir in garlic and pepper and cook for a couple of minutes.
3. Add 2 cups of water and meat bouillon cubes.
4. Close the lid. Select 'Manual' and set the timer for 5 minutes.
5. When the timer goes off, let the pressure release naturally.
6. Mix together cornmeal in remaining water. Add into the instant pot.
7. Press 'Sauté' button. Press 'Adjust' button twice. Simmer for a few minutes.
8. To make plantain mash: Place plantains in the microwave and microwave on High for 4-5 minutes. Peel and slice

plantains and transfer into a blender. Add coconut milk. Blend for 35-40 seconds or until smooth.

9. Transfer into a saucepan. Add butter and Parmesan cheese and stir. Place over medium heat and simmer until smooth and well combined. Taste and add more salt if necessary.

Servings: 2

Ingredients:

- 4 ounces Fideo noodles
- 1 clove garlic, minced
- ½ ripe avocado, peeled, pitted, sliced, to garnish (optional)
- 1 ½ table-spoons vegetable oil
- 1 plum tomato, halved, deseeded
- 1 small white onion, chopped
- 4 cups homemade chicken broth
- Salt to taste

Method:

1. Puree the tomato and set aside.
2. Place a saucepan over medium heat. Add oil. When the oil is heated, add noodles and sauté until it begins to become brown. Some noodles will be browner than the rest.
3. Add blended tomato, garlic and onion and mix until the noodles are well coated.
4. Pour broth and salt and mix well.
5. When it begins to boil, lower heat and cover with a lid. Simmer for 7-9 minutes.
6. Ladle into soup bowls and serve garnished with avocado.

Servings: for 3-4 people

Ingredients:

- 24 ounces of goat meat
- 1 table-spoon of curry powder
- 1 table-spoon of white vinegar
- 1 stalk of scallion, chopped
- ½ medium sized onion, chopped
- ½ tea-spoon of ginger, chopped
- 2 cloves of garlic, chopped
- ¼ of hot pepper, chopped
- 1 tea-spoon of fresh thyme, chopped
- ½ tea-spoon of salt
- ½ tea-spoon of black pepper
- 2 cups of water, boiling
- 2 table-spoons of vegetable oil
- ½ of a medium-sized carrot, sliced
- ½ large Irish potato, diced
- 2 allspice berries, whole and crushed

Method:

1. Cut the meat into pieces that are bite-sized then wash using a mix of vinegar and water.
2. Place the meat in a bowl; add half a table-spoon of the curry powder, onion, ginger, scallion, thyme, black pepper, hot pepper, salt, and garlic to the meat and rub all of these seasonings properly into the pieces. Cover the boule and let it infuse for 2 hours.
3. Place a skillet over medium heat, and heat some oil in it. Add in the rest of the curry powder and also the meat you have marinated. Let it sear then carefully turn the pieces of the meat and add the boiling water.
4. Cover the skillet and let it simmer for one hour and twenty minutes or until the meat turns tender.

5. Once that is done, add the potato and let it cook for another
    5 minutes.
6. Lastly, fold in the allspice berries and carrot and give it a
    final cooking of 7 minutes.
7. Serve hot with rice.

Servings:

Ingredients:

- ½ pound dry black eyed beans of green beans, soaked in water overnight
- 1 clove garlic, crushed
- 2-3 table-spoons finely chopped green bell pepper
- 1 table-spoon oil
- ½ cup cassava flour
- ¼ pound bacon
- 1 medium onion, chopped
- A handful fresh cilantro, chopped
- 1 tea-spoon paprika
- Salt to taste

Method:

1. Drain and rinse the beans and place in the instant pot. Pour enough water to cover it.
2. Close the lid. Select 'Manual' button and set the timer for 15 minutes.
3. When the timer geos off, let the pressure release naturally. Transfer the beans into a bowl.
4. Wipe the pot clean.
5. Select 'Sauté' button. Add the bacon and cook until it becomes crisp. Remove bacon with a slotted spoon and place on your cutting board. When cool enough to handle, chop into smaller pieces.
6. Add the onions and sauté until translucent. Add the garlic and stir.
7. Add cilantro, green pepper and paprika and mix well. Drain the beans and add into the pot. Sprinkle salt and mix well.
8. Press 'Adjust' button twice and simmer for 5-7 minutes.
9. Stir in cassava flour and bacon. Simmer for 4-5 minutes and serve.

Servings: 2

Ingredients:

<u>For salad:</u>

- 1 fajita size flour tortilla, halved, cut into ½ inch strips
- Salt to taste
- ½ pound 93% lean ground turkey
- ½ tea-spoon ground cumin
- ½ head romaine lettuce, chopped
- 5.5 ounces canned Mexican style corn, drained
- 1 small ripe avocado, peeled, pitted, chopped
- ¼ cup low fat sharp cheddar cheese, shredded
- 1 tea-spoon extra-virgin olive oil, divided
- Pepper powder to taste
- ½ table-spoon chili powder
- ¼ tea-spoon garlic powder
- 7.5 ounces canned low sodium black beans, rinsed, drained
- 1 cup cherry tomato, halved
- ½ cup cilantro, chopped
- 1 green onion, thinly sliced
- Cooking spray

<u>For yogurt salsa dressing:</u>

- 2 table-spoons plain nonfat Greek yogurt
- 2 table-spoons salsa

Method:

1. Adjust the frame in the middle of the oven.
2. Grease a rimmed baking sheet with nonstick cooking spray.
3. Spread the tortilla strips in the center of the baking sheet. Brush with ½ tea-spoon oil. Season with salt and pepper.

Toss well. Spread it all over the baking sheet, in a single layer.

4. Bake in a preheated oven at 435° F for 8- 10 minutes or until crisp. Flip sides halfway through baking. Remove from the oven and cool. Set aside to garnish.
5. Place a nonstick skillet over medium high heat. Add remaining oil. When the oil is heated, add turkey, garlic powder, pepper, salt, chili powder and cumin powder and mix well.
6. Break the meat simultaneously as it cooks. Cook until the meat is tender.
7. Add salsa and yogurt into a bowl and mix well.
8. Add romaine lettuce into a serving bowl. Add meat mixture and rest of the ingredients. Toss well.
9. Divide into 2 bowls. Top with tortilla strips and serve.

Servings: 2-3

Ingredients:

- 2-3 whole medium or small sized snappers – or Parrot, Grount, or Goat Fish – Clean and scale, leave the tail and head on
- ¾ tea-spoon of pepper
- ¾ tea-spoon of salt
- 2 cloves of garlic
- White vinegar
- Cooking oil
- 1 scotch bonnet pepper
- 1 onion
- 5 pimento/allspice seeds

Method:

1. Make sure the fish is cleaned and scaled properly. Wash it with water and then give it a wash with a mixture of water and vinegar.
2. Once washed, dry them using paper towels; then place them on a plate and set it aside.
3. On each side of each fish – cut some small but deep gashes.
4. Take the salt and pepper and rub them into these gashes and all over the fish. Then place them back on the plate.
5. Heat some oil in a frying pan to shallow fry the fish – take enough oil to partially submerge the fish. Do not submerge it completely.
6. Add one clove of garlic to the pan and turn the heat to high. After 35 seconds or so, remove the garlic from the pan.
7. Next, place the fish very carefully in the hot. Do not overcrowd the pan, just place as many as can be accommodated by the pan.
8. Fry until it is crisp on one side then turn it to the other side carefully and fry until crisp. Bring the heat down as and when required.

9. Once done, transfer them to a plate that has been lined with paper towels.
10. Take the scotch bonnet pepper and onion – slice both of them.
11. Add the sliced scotch bonnet pepper, pimento, and onions in a small sized pot, add in some vinegar, make sure you add enough to submerge everything else in the pot. Boil everything for around 3-4 minutes. Be careful as it boils – avoid letting it overheat as it could make your eyes burn.
12. Pour the spicy vinegar mix over the fried fish to induce a spicy and hot flavor.

Servings:

Ingredients:

- 10 pequi fruits, rinsed
- 1 medium onion, finely chopped
- 1-2 red cherry peppers
- 1-2 green onions, thinly sliced
- Salt to taste
- 1 cup white rice, rinsed
- 4 table-spoons olive oil
- 2 cups hot water

Method:

1. Make incisions on the outer surface of the pequis.
2. Select 'Sauté' button. Add oil. When the oil is heated, add pequi and onion and sauté for 9-10 minutes.
3. Add rice and sauté for a few minutes until rice turns opaque.
4. Add salt, cherry pepper and water.
5. Close the lid. Select 'Rice' button.
6. When the rice cycle completes, sprinkle onions on top and fluff with a fork.

Servings: 4

Ingredients:

<u>For dressing:</u>

- ¼ cup plain, nonfat yogurt
- ½ tea-spoon honey
- A large pinch cumin
- ½ table-spoon lime juice
- ¼ tea-spoon paprika

<u>For salad:</u>

- 2 ears corn, shucked, remove kernels (about 1 ½ cups kernels)
- ½ cup canned or cooked black beans, drained, rinsed
- 2 table-spoons extra-virgin olive oil
- 1 small red bell pepper, deseeded, chopped
- ¼ cup cilantro, finely chopped
- 1 large jalapeño chili or to taste, finely sliced
- 1 small red onion, peeled, chopped
- 1 table-spoon lime juice
- 1 small clove garlic, minced
- ¼ cup cotija cheese, shredded
- Sea salt to taste

Method:

1. To make dressing: Add all the ingredients of the dressing into a bowl and whisk well. Cover and set aside for a while for the flavors to set in.
2. Place a nonstick skillet over medium heat. Add oil. When the oil is heated, add garlic and corn and cook until the

corn slightly begins to become brown. Stir frequently. Transfer into a bowl.

3. Add lime juice, black beans, onion, cheese, red pepper and cilantro and toss well.
4. Divide salad into serving plates. Divide the dressing and drizzle on top.
5. It can be served cold or warm. You can also serve over tacos or with chips.

Servings: 3

Ingredients:

- 3 chicken breast halves, boneless and cut into bite-sized chunks
- ½ cup of water
- Juice of 2 limes
- ¼ tea-spoon of ground nutmeg
- 1 tea-spoon of ground allspice
- ½ tea-spoon of brown sugar
- ½ tea-spoon of salt
- 1 tea-spoon of thyme, dried
- ¾ tea-spoon of black ground pepper
- 1 onion, chopped
- 1 table-spoon of vegetable oil
- ½ tea-spoon of ground ginger
- 3/4cup of green onions, chopped
- 1 habanero pepper, chopped
- 3 cloves of garlic, chopped

Method:

1. Cut the chicken into bite-sized chunks and place them in a bowl. Drizzle the lime juice over it and mix it well enough to coat all the chunks in the lime juice. Set it aside.
2. Add the nutmeg, allspice, salt, thyme, brown sugar, black pepper, vegetable oil, and ginger to a food processor and blend. Then add in the chopped green onions, chopped onion, chopped habanero, and garlic and blend until everything is properly combined and almost smooth.
3. Save a third of the mixture for later use and add the rest to the bowl of chicken. Mix it well and make sure all the chunks of chicken are properly coated in the marinade. Cover the bowl and place it in the refrigerator for around 2 hours, minimum.

4. Once that is done, heat a grill pan with some oil. Place the chicken on it and allow it to cook slowly. Turn the chunks frequently and baste them often using the marinade you have saved. Cook until the chicken has cooked through.

Servings: 3

Ingredients:

- 2 table-spoons olive oil
- ¾ cup rice
- 5 ounces canned Italian plum tomatoes, drained, chopped
- A handful cilantro to garnish
- 1 onion, finely chopped
- 1 ½ cups hot chicken broth
- Salt to taste
- 1 tomato, cut into wedges, to serve

Method:

1. Select 'Sauté' Add oil. When the oil is heated, add onions and cook until translucent.
2. Add rice and sauté until well coated.
3. Stir in the tomatoes, broth and salt. Press 'Cancel' button.
4. Close the lid. Select 'Rice' button.
5. When the rice cycle is completed, fluff with a fork.
6. Sprinkle cilantro and tomatoes on top and serve.

Servings: 2

Ingredients:

- 6.4 ounces lean ground beef (85% to 89%)
- 3 green onions, separate the white and green parts, chopped
- 1 small tomato, chopped
- 1 ½ ounces canned olives, sliced
- 3 table-spoons fat free Greek or plain yogurt
- 1 tea-spoon chili powder
- 1/3 head romaine lettuce, chopped
- 1/3 avocado, peeled, pitted, chopped
- ½ cup fat free cheese like cheddar or Monterey Jack cheese
- 3 table-spoons salsa

Method:

1. Place a skillet over medium heat. Add beef, white of onion, chili powder, and pepper and salt. Sauté until beef is cooked. Turn off the heat. Cover and set aside if you would like a warm salad or cool completely and chill in the refrigerator if you like chilled salad.
2. Add lettuce, avocado, tomato, greens of the onion and olives into a bowl and toss well. Add the cooked beef and cheese and stir.
3. Divide the salad into serving plates. Drizzle yogurt and salsa on top and serve.

Beef Patties

Servings: 5-6

Ingredients:

<u>Piecrust:</u>

- 2 cups of all-purpose flour
- ¼ table-spoon of salt
- 2 ½ ounces of shortening
- 1 table-spoon of sugar
- ¼ tea-spoon of turmeric
- ½ table-spoon of cider vinegar
- 2 ½ ounces of butter
- ½ cup of iced water

<u>Beef filling:</u>

- 8 ounces of ground beef
- ½ tea-spoon of garlic, granulated
- ¼ of a medium sized onion, chopped
- ½ tea-spoon of paprika
- ½ tea-spoon of curry powder
- ¼ tea-spoon of allspice powder
- ½ tea-spoon of white pepper
- ½ thyme, dried
- 1-2 green onions, chopped
- ¼ tea-spoon or more or less of salt
- 1 table-spoon of parsley, fresh and chopped
- ¼ tea-spoon of chili powder
- 3 table-spoons of breadcrumbs
- ½ tea-spoon of chicken bouillon powder
- ¼ scotch bonnet pepper, chopped – optional
- 1 egg white for brushing

Method:

1. Add the flour, sugar, salt, and turmeric to a food processor and blend until everything is properly combined. This can also be done by hand.
2. Add in the shortening, vinegar, butter and the water in installments. Keep pulsing until the mixture is properly combined and forms enough into a dough that holds shape like a ball.
3. Lightly flour a working surface and place the dough on it then roll the dough out.
4. Once rolled out, put it in the fridge for about 30 minutes or until it is ready to be used.
5. Using a bowl or glass, cut out as many circles as possible. Once you have cut all of the dough away into circles, refrigerate them for around 30 minutes or until they are ready to be sued.
6. Now, as they rest in the refrigerator, prepare your beef pie filling by placing a saucepan over medium heat and adding a table-spoon of oil. Once it's hot, add in the onions, paprika, garlic, curry powder, thyme, white pepper, allspice, chili powder and the bouillon. Allow it to simmer for around 2 minutes.
7. Once done, add in the ground beef, along with the breadcrumbs and let it cook for around 10 minutes or minutes. Keep stirring it to prevent it from burning. Add ¼ cup of water.
8. Next, add the parsley and green onions, give it a taste and adjust the pepper and salt seasoning.
9. Take it off the heat and allow it to cool.
10. Assembly – once the filling has cooled down completely, scoop out one table-spoon of the beef filling; place it in the middle of each circle of dough. Brush the edges of the circle with some egg white and fold the circle over and twist it, using your fingers, keep twisting around the edges until they are fully closed. Be gentle and properly seal the edges of the meat pie.
11. You can also seal the dough circles by pressing the edges down with a fork.

12. Preheat the oven to 385F.
13. Prepare a baking sheet by lining it with parchment paper.
14. Place the pies carefully on the prepared baking sheet.
15. Bake for 30 minutes.
16. Serve warm. Enjoy!

Servings: 6

Ingredients:

- 1 ½ table-spoons vegetable oil
- 3 cups hot water
- 1 ½ cups long grain rice
- ¼ tea-spoon salt

Method:

1. Select 'Sauté' button. Add oil. When the oil is heated, add rice and sauté until it is golden brown in color. Stir frequently.
2. Add water and salt and stir. Press 'Cancel' button.
3. Close the lid. Select 'Rice' button.
4. When the rice cycle is completed, fluff with a fork.

Servings: 4

Ingredients:

- 6 table-spoons whole wheat flour
- Salt to taste
- 1 table-spoon + 1 tea-spoon extra-virgin olive oil
- Salt to taste
- 6 table-spoons corn
- 3 table-spoons pickled jalapeños
- 1 large egg white
- 2 large eggs
- 6 table-spoons low fat milk
- Freshly ground pepper to taste
- 6 table-spoons all-purpose flour
- 1 table-spoon cold butter, chopped into small pieces
- 1-2 table-spoons ice water
- 1 cup onion, chopped
- 1 table-spoon water
- ¼ cup cherry tomatoes, quartered
- ¼ cup Jack cheese, shredded
- 3 table-spoons sour cream

Method:

1. To make crust: Add wheat flour, salt and all-purpose flour into a bowl and mix well.
2. Add butter and mix with your fingers until the butter is well mixed into the flour mixture.
3. Stir in 2 table-spoons sour cream and oil and mix with a fork until well combined.
4. Add iced water and mix until the mixture is soft and well combined. Add a table-spoon of water if necessary. Knead the dough for a couple of minutes.

5. Shape the dough into a circle. Cover the bowl with cling wrap and chill for 1 hour.
6. Grease a small 6-inch pie pan with cooking spray.
7. Place a skillet over high heat. Add oil. When the oil is heated, add onion and salt and sauté until it begins to become brown.
8. Add water and lower heat. Cook until onions turn golden brown. Turn off the heat.
9. Place a sheet of parchment paper over your countertop. Place the dough on the parchment paper.
10. Roll the dough with a rolling pin into a circle of about 8-9 inches.
11. Carefully invert the pie pan on the rolled dough in the center.
12. Invert again the entire thing along with the parchment paper (hold one hand below the parchment paper, underneath the rolled dough and one hand on the pie pan).
13. Carefully remove the paper and press the rolled dough on to the pie pan on the bottom as well as the sides. Crimp the excess rolled dough along the edges.
14. Spread the onions over the dough in the pan. Spread corn over it followed by tomatoes and jalapeños.
15. Sprinkle cheese on top.
16. Add eggs, whites, sour cream, milk, pepper, 1-table-spoon sour cream and salt into a bowl and whisk well.
17. Pour over the vegetables in the pie pan.
18. Bake in a preheated oven at 385° F for 30-40 minutes or set and firm in the center.
19. Remove from the oven and cool for 15 minutes.
20. Cut into 4 wedges and serve.

Steamed Fish

Servings: 4

Ingredients:

- 4 red snappers, whole, scaled and cleaned
- 2 tea-spoons of fresh thyme, chopped
- 2 whole lemons
- 2 medium-sized onions, sliced
- 2 tea-spoons of minced garlic
- 2 tea-spoons of paprika
- 1 tea-spoon of grated ginger
- 1 tea-spoon of allspice
- 2 medium-sized tomatoes, diced
- 4 green onions, chopped
- 2 bell peppers, sliced
- 2 hot peppers, or as per taste
- 4 cups fish stock, or more or less
- 4 or more cups of chopped vegetables – chayote, potatoes, carrots
- 2 tea-spoon bouillon powder or cubes – optional
- Salt and pepper to taste
- 4 table-spoons of butter
- Black pepper to taste

Method:

1. Clean and scale the fish. Rinse it then drain it carefully and pat it dry using paper towels. Once done, rub it using lemon.
2. Take a large bowl or shallow pan and place the fish in it and season it with ginger, half of the garlic, salt, black pepper, and half of the thyme. Turn the fish and rub all the seasonings all over to make sure they are coated well.
3. Place the dish in the refrigerator and let it marinate for thirty minutes or even overnight.
4. Add 2 or more table-spoons of oil to a large skillet and heat it. Add in the onion, garlic, thyme, allspice, and paprika.

5. Add in the veggies and add the ones that have the longest cooking time first – like potatoes. Then add in the fish stock and bring everything to a boil. Once it starts boiling, cover it then allow it to simmer for about 5 minutes.
6. Carefully place the fish in the boiling stock and add in the green onion, tomato, and hot pepper.
7. Spoon the stock on top of the fish then cover and allow it to steam over medium heat for around 5-6 minutes or until the meat is tender on each side – cooking time may vary depending on how thick the fish is.
8. Add the butter over the fish before you take it off the stove.
9. Serve with rice or crackers.

Servings: 6

Ingredients:

- 3 table-spoons olive oil
- 6 cloves garlic, minced
- 3 tea-spoons dried oregano
- 3 cups vegetable stock
- 1 ½ cups cooked chickpeas
- 1/3 cup fresh parsley, chopped
- Salt to taste
- Pepper to taste
- 2 onions, diced
- 1 tea-spoon turmeric powder
- 1 ½ cups brown rice
- 1 ½ cups sweet corn
- Juice of a lime
- Zest of a lime
- 1/3 cup fresh cilantro, chopped

Method:

1. Select 'Sauté' Add oil. When the oil is heated, add onions and cook until translucent. Add garlic and sauté until fragrant. Add oregano, turmeric and rice.
2. Add rice and sauté until well coated.
3. Add stock and stir. Press 'Cancel' button.
4. Close the lid. Select 'Rice' button.
5. When the rice cycle is completed, add rest of the ingredients and mix well.
6. Serve hot.

Servings: 3 (2 tacos each)

Ingredients:

- 1 tea-spoon olive oil
- ¼ tea-spoons dried oregano
- 1 jalapeno pepper, seeded, minced
- ½ table-spoon low sodium soy sauce
- ½ package seitan (from an 8 ounce package, wheat gluten), finely chopped
- 6 taco shells
- 1 small onion, chopped
- 2 cloves garlic, minced
- ½ table-spoon dry sherry
- 7.5 ounces canned black beans, with its liquid
- ¼ tea-spoon black pepper
- 1 cup shredded romaine lettuce
- Avocado salsa to serve

Method:

1. Place a nonstick skillet over medium heat. Add oil. When the oil is heated, add onion, garlic, jalapeño and oregano and sauté for 5-6 minutes.
2. Add dry sherry, soy sauce, beans, and seitan. Mix well. Cook until nearly dry.
3. Add pepper and stir.
4. Follow the directions on the package and make the taco shells.
5. Divide the filling among the taco shells. Top with lettuce and avocado salsa.

Servings: 10-12

Ingredients:

- 2 small whole chickens, cut down to portions
- 6-8 stalks of scallions, chopped
- 2 large tomatoes
- 2 large onions, chopped
- 2 scotch bonnet peppers, chopped
- 4 cloves of garlic, chopped
- ½ cup of lime juice
- 2 medium-sized carrots, finely chopped
- 5-6 sprigs of fresh thyme or 3-4 tea-spoons of dried thyme
- 4 table-spoons of soy sauce
- 1-2 tea-spoons of allspice, cracked
- 4 cups of coconut milk, unsweetened
- 2 table-spoons of coconut oil
- 4 tea-spoons of cornstarch, or 1 table-spoon of flour

Method:

1. Pour the lime juice over the chicken you have cut down to portions. Rub the lime juice all over the chicken and make sure it gets an even coating. Drain out the excess juice.
2. Take a large bowl and combine the scallion, tomatoes, onions, thyme, soy sauce, allspice, pepper, and garlic along with the pieces of chicken. Cover it and let it marinate for around 1 hour.
3. Heat some oil in a large saucepan. As you take the pieces of chicken out of the marinade, shake the seasonings of each individual piece. Reserve this marinade to be used for sauce.
4. Brown the chicken lightly over high heat, do it a few pieces of chicken at a time. Once a batch is done, place them on a plate.
5. Drain the excess oil off the chicken and place them back in the pan. Add the marinade on top of the chicken followed by the carrots.

6. Give everything a nice stir then allow it to cook on medium heat for around 10 minutes.
7. Mix the coconut milk and flour then pour it into the stew, keep stirring continuously.
8. Bring the heat down to low and then allow it to cook for 25 minutes or until the chicken is tender.
9. Serve hot, and enjoy!

Servings: 4

Ingredients:

- 2 table-spoons butter
- 1 small onion, chopped
- ½ cup dry white wine
- 4-6 hearts of palm, sliced
- 2 table-spoons flat leaf parsley, chopped
- 1 tea-spoon salt
- 2 table-spoons olive oil
- 10 ounces Arborio rice
- 6 cups vegetable stock
- 2 table-spoons Parmesan cheese, freshly grated
- 2 table-spoons cold butter
- ½ tea-spoon white pepper

Method:

1. Select 'Sauté' Add oil. When the oil is heated, add onions and cook until translucent.
2. Add rice and sauté for 3 minutes. Add white wine. Cook for a couple of minutes and add broth.
3. Close the lid. Select 'Rice' button. Press 'Cancel' button.
4. When the rice cycle completes, add hearts of palm and stir. Stir in butter, cheese, salt, pepper and parsley.

Servings: 2

Ingredients:

- 4 ounces chicken breasts, skinless boneless, trimmed
- Salt to taste
- Freshly ground pepper to taste
- 1 table-spoon nonfat plain yogurt
- ½ table-spoon fresh cilantro, chopped
- A large pinch ground cumin
- 2 whole wheat flour tortillas
- 1 small tomato, thinly sliced

Method:

1. Place chicken in a glass bowl. Season with salt and pepper. Drizzle lime juice. Set aside for 10 minutes.
2. Add yogurt, cilantro, cumin, sour cream, salt and jalapeño into a bowl. Whisk well.
3. Grease a baking sheet with a little oil. Place chicken on the baking sheet.
4. Broil in a preheated oven for 4-5 minutes.
5. Add onion and stir. Broil for a few more minutes until the chicken is not pink anymore and cooked through.
6. Warm the tortillas following the instructions on the package.
7. Spread the tortillas on your countertop. Place chicken, lettuce leaves, onions and tomato slices.
8. Drizzle yogurt mixture on top. Roll and serve right away.

Servings: 2

Ingredients:

- 2 pork loin chops, boneless
- ½ table-spoon of orange juice
- ½ table-spoon of soy sauce
- ½ table-spoon of olive oil
- 1-2 green onions, minced
- 2 cloves of garlic, minced
- ½ tea-spoon of allspice, ground
- ¼ tea-spoon of salt
- ½ tea-spoon of dried thyme
- ¼ tea-spoon of ginger
- ¼ tea-spoon of pepper
- A pinch of cayenne

Method:

1. Prepare the pork chops by slashing off some of the fat around the chops – slash at intervals. This is to remove the excess fat while keeping just enough for it to cook in.
2. Take a bowl and add in the salt, soy sauce, pepper, orange juice and oil. Stir everything up.
3. Add in the garlic, green onion, thyme, allspice, ginger, cayenne, and thyme. Mix well.
4. Take this mixture and rub it on both sides of the chops. Make sure to rub the seasonings and spices in properly. Let it rest for 1 hour to enhance the flavors.
5. Preheat the oven to 370F.
6. Lightly grease a roasting pan. Place the marinated chops in it.
7. Roast and turn the chops halfway through.
8. Roast until the chops have browned and the juices they give off are running clear when you pierce it with a knife or fork. This will take about 20 minutes.
9. Serve hot, and enjoy!

Servings: 3

Ingredients:

- 2 ½ cups chicken stock
- 2 table-spoons unsalted butter
- 1 clove garlic, chopped
- 3 ounces smoked back bacon, diced
- 3 ounces smoked sausage or chorizo, finely sliced
- 3 ounces pork loin steaks
- 1 ¼ cups Arborio rice or any other short grain rice
- 3 table-spoons Parmesan cheese, grated + extra to serve
- 2 kale or savoy cabbage leaves
- ½ table-spoon corn or sunflower oil
- 1 small onion, chopped
- ½ cup dry white wine
- ½ can red kidney beans, drained, rinsed
- 1 small red chili, deseeded, finely chopped + extra to garnish

Method:

1. Select 'Sauté' button. Add oil and half the butter. When butter melts, add onion, garlic, bacon and sausage and sauté until onions are pink.
2. Add rice and sauté for 3 minutes. Add white wine. Cook for a couple of minutes and add 2 cups stock. Press 'Cancel' button.
3. Close the lid. Select 'Rice' button.
4. When the rice cycle completes, stir in beans and chili. Stir and add remaining stock.
5. Tear one kale leaf and add into the instant pot. Add remaining salt, pepper, butter and cheese and stir.
6. Meanwhile, sprinkle salt and pepper over the pork. Grill on a preheated grill. When cool enough to handle, slice the pork.
7. Chop the other kale leaf finely and place on individual serving plates.

8. Serve risotto over kale. Sprinkle chili and Parmesan cheese
    and serve.

Servings: 2

Ingredients:

- 1 small sweet yellow pepper, chopped
- 1 tea-spoon olive oil
- 1 table-spoon mayonnaise
- 6 table-spoons Mexican cheese blend, shredded
- 1 small green bell pepper, chopped
- 4 slices rye bread
- ½ cup fresh salsa, drained
- 1 table-spoon butter, softened

Method:

1. Place a skillet over medium heat. Add oil. When the oil is heated, add peppers and sauté until tender.
2. Apply mayonnaise on 3 slices of bread.
3. Divide the pepper mixture over it. Divide and spread salsa and cheese over the peppers.
4. Cover with the remaining 3 slices of bread.
5. Brush butter on the outside of the sandwiches.
6. Place a skillet over medium heat. Cook the sandwiches on both the sides until golden brown.
7. Cut into desired shape and serve.

Curry Chicken

Servings: 4

Ingredients:

- 24 ounces of chicken
- Onion powder, as per taste
- 2 ounces of curry powder
- 1 tea-spoon of salt
- 2 table-spoons of oil
- 1-2 tea-spoons of garlic powder
- 1 table-spoon of vinegar
- 1 medium-sized potato, diced
- ¼ to ½ tea-spoon of black pepper - optional
- ¼ cup of water
- 1 sprig of thyme – optional

Method:

1. Slice the chicken into 4 or more pieces. Wash the chicken with a mixture of water and vinegar.
2. Place the chicken in a bowl and add in all of the ingredients.
3. Rub the spices and seasonings into the chicken thoroughly until the powders are wet and stick to the chicken properly.
4. Place a skillet over high heat and heat the cooking oil along with a table-spoon of curry powder, until the powder changes in color.
5. Add in the pieces of chicken to the skillet and reduce the heat to medium, instantly followed by water.
6. Add in the potato and cover the pot. Allow it to simmer.
7. Give everything in the pot a nice stir and taste to check the salt and seasoning of the gravy.
8. Make whatever adjustments required.
9. Optional – add in the black pepper and thyme.
10. Let it simmer and cook until the chicken is tender.
11. Once done, remove the chicken pieces out of the skillet and into a bowl.

12. Turn the heat to high and allow the gravy to cook a bit to thicken it.
13. Once it has reduced considerably to a desired consistency, turn the heat off, and add the chicken back.
14. Serve hot, and enjoy!

Servings: 6

Ingredients:

<u>For salsa:</u>

- 2 medium ripe mangoes, peeled, pitted, finely chopped
- 1 large chili pepper, deseeded, minced
- Juice of a large orange
- 1/3 cup mint leaves, chopped
- 1 ½ tea-spoons dark brown sugar

<u>For risotto:</u>

- 3 cups coconut milk
- 4 ½ table-spoons coconut oil
- 1 ½ cups Arborio rice
- Freshly ground pepper to taste
- Salt to taste
- ¾ cup toasted coconut flakes, unsweetened
- Lime wedges to serve
- 3 cups vegetable broth
- 2 medium onions, finely chopped
- ¾ cup cachaca
- 1 ½ pounds crab meat, canned or refrigerated, gently pulled apart
- Zest of 3 limes, grated

Method:

1. To make mango salsa: Add all the ingredients of mango salsa into a bowl and mix until well combined. Cover and set sideways for a while for the tastes to set in.
2. Select 'Sauté' Add oil. When the oil is heated, add onions and cook until translucent.

3. Add rice and sauté for 3 minutes. Add. Cook for a couple of minutes and add broth. Press 'Cancel' button.
4. Add coconut milk and broth into a saucepan. Place saucepan over medium heat. Pour into the instant pot and stir.
5. Close the lid. Select 'Rice' button. When the rice cycle completes, add rest of the ingredients and stir.
6. Serve in bowls. Place mango salsa on top and serve.

Servings: 2

Ingredients:

- ½ red apple, peeled, cored, chopped
- 1 small banana, sliced
- 1 apricot, deseeded, chopped
- ½ pear or peach, peeled, chopped
- ½ orange, peeled, separated into segments, deseeded
- 2 cups milk
- Sugar to taste
- Ice cubes, as required

Method:

1. Add milk, apple, pear, banana and orange into a blender.
2. Blend until smooth.
3. Pour into tall chilled glasses and serve.

Servings: 2

Ingredients:

- 8 ounces of beef oxtail, cut down to pieces
- 1 green onion, sliced thinly
- 1 -sized onion, chopped
- 1 clove of garlic, minced
- ½ of a scotch bonnet pepper, chopped
- ½ tea-spoon of fresh ginger, minced
- 1 table-spoon of soy sauce
- 1 sprig of thyme, fresh and chopped
- ¼ tea-spoon of salt
- 1 table-spoon of vegetable oil
- ½ tea-spoon of black pepper
- ¾ cup of water
- ½ tea-spoon of allspice berries, whole
- ½ cup of fava beans, drained
- 2 table-spoons of water
- ½ table-spoon of cornstarch

Method:

1. Take the meat in a medium-sized bowl and add in the green onion, scotch bonnet pepper, garlic, onion, thyme, soy sauce, pepper, and salt.
2. Toss the contents of the bowl until everything is properly combined and evenly coated.
3. Heat a skillet over medium to high heat and add in the vegetable oil. Add the meat mixture to the pan and allow the oxtail to brown.
4. Let it brown all over, it will take around.
5. Put everything in a pressure cooker, and add in ¾ cup of water.
6. Cook in the pressure cooker for around 25 minutes.

7. Once done, remove the pressure cooker from the heat, and then very carefully take the lid off.
8. Add in the beans along with the allspice berries and let it come to a simmer on medium to high heat.
9. Mix the cornstarch with the 3 table-spoons of water and add it to the simmering contents, and keep stirring.
10. Stir and cook for a few minutes more until the sauce thickens up and the beans become tender.
11. Serve hot, and enjoy!

Servings: 5-6

Ingredients:

- ¼ cup yuca flour (manioc flour)
- 1 ¼ cups yellow cornmeal, medium or coarsely ground
- 3 table-spoons olive oil + extra to grease
- 1 small green bell pepper, finely chopped
- 1 small red bell pepper, finely chopped
- Salt to taste
- Pepper to taste
- 6.5 ounces hearts of palm, drained, chopped
- 6 ounces tomato sauce
- 1 cup frozen peas, divided
- 1 medium onion, finely chopped
- ½ cup scallions, finely chopped
- 1 bay leaf
- 2 large cloves garlic, minced
- 1 cup chicken stock
- ¾ pound small or medium shrimp, peeled, deveined
- ¼ cup green olives, finely chopped
- 2 eggs, hard boiled, peeled, cut into slices
- 4 large shrimp, peeled, deveined, to garnish

For sauce:

- 1 table-spoon olive oil
- 1 small jalapeño, deseeded, minced
- ¼ cup tomato sauce
- ¼ cup fresh cilantro, chopped
- 3 table-spoons finely chopped onion
- 1 large ripe tomato, chopped
- Salt to taste

Method:

1. Add corn meal and yuca flour into a bowl and stir until well combined.
2. Select 'Sauté' Add oil. When the oil is heated, add onions and cook until translucent.
3. Add garlic and sauté for a few seconds until fragrant.
4. Add bell peppers and bay leaf. Stir in stock, hearts of palm and tomato sauce. Press 'Cancel' button.
5. Close the lid. Select 'Manual' button and set the timer for 2 minutes.
6. When the timer goes off, let the pressure release naturally for 4 minutes after which, quick release excess pressure.
7. Sprinkle salt and pepper over shrimp and add into the instant pot. Add about ¾ cup peas.
8. Select 'Sauté' button and press 'Adjust' button twice. Let it simmer for 5 minutes. Discard the bay leaf.
9. Add green olives, scallions and stir. Stir in the flour mixture. Stir constantly until cooked through.
10. Taste and adjust the salt if necessary. Press 'Cancel' button. Close the lid and set aside.
11. Place the large shrimp on a greased baking sheet. Sprinkle salt and pepper over it.
12. Place rack about 5 inches away from the heating element.
13. Place shrimp in the oven and broil for a few minutes until shrimp curls and is pink in color.
14. Grease a small Bundt pan and place egg slices, remaining peas and shrimp on it. Spread the cooked flour mixture over it. Press lightly. Cover with foil and let it sit for some time.
15. Meanwhile, make the sauce as follows: Place a skillet over medium heat. Add oil. When the oil is heated, add onion and jalapeño and cook until onions are translucent.
16. Add rest of the ingredients except cilantro and mix well. Cook for 2-3 minutes. Turn off the heat. Add cilantro and stir.
17. Invert on to a plate. Serve with salsa.

Servings: 2

Ingredients:

- 2 slices pineapple
- Juice of ½ lemon
- Juice of an orange
- 1 ½ bananas, peeled, sliced
- ¼ cup chilled sugar syrup

Method:

1. Add pineapple, banana, sugar syrup, lemon juice and orange juice into a blender.
2. Blend until smooth.
3. Pour into tall chilled glasses and serve garnished with an orange slice or lemon slice.

Servings: 4-6

Ingredients:

- 10-12 medium sized cremini mushrooms (sliced into strips)
- 4 cloves garlic (finely minced)
- 3 table-spoons of berbere spice
- 3 table-spoons oil
- 1 2-inch piece of ginger (peeled then finely minced)
- 1 table-spoon water
- ½ an onion (julienned)
- ½ medium-large tomato (cut into wedges)
- salt, pepper, dried or fresh parsley

Method:

1. First, heat the oil in a pan or skillet over medium heat. Add the onion, mixing to coat with the oil. Boil just till the onions starts attractive tender (1-2 minutes).
2. Add the sliced mushrooms. Fry until the burgeons start turning color (2-3 minutes), then add the tomato slices. Add the minced garlic and ginger.
3. Stirring composed the berbere interest and water, until you form a thick paste. Stir the paste into the mushroom mixture, until everything is evenly coated.
4. Add a pinch of salt, pinch of pepper, and a generous pinch of parsley. Cook for 12-15 minutes until the mushrooms are fully cooked.
5. Serve with injera.

Melon Frullato

Servings: 2

Ingredients:

- ½ melon (honeydew or watermelon or cantaloupe), peeled, cubed, deseeded
- Juice of ½ lemon
- 2 tea-spoons sugar
- 1 tea-spoon liquor of your choice (optional)
- Ice cubes, as required
- 2 cups dry Chablis

Method:

1. Add melon, lemon juice, sugar, liquor, ice cubes and Chablis into a blender.
2. Blend until smooth.
3. Pour into tall chilled glasses and serve garnished with a melon slice.

Servings: 2-4

Ingredients:

- 1 lb. ground lean beef
- 4 cup water (boiled)
- 1 tea-spoon garlic precipitate
- 1 cup onion (thinly chopped)
- ½ cup ghee
- ¼ cup white wine (if preferred)
- ¼ tea-spoon cardamom powder (korerima)
- ¼ ginger powder
- ¼ tea-spoon turmeric or curry
- ¼ tea-spoon white pepper powder
- salt and pepper to taste

Method:

1. Sauté the onion in medium pot using one cup of boiled water by adding two table-spoon each time until the onion is soft and golden brown.
2. In the cooked onion, add one cup boiled water, ghee, garlic, ginger, wine and turmeric. Cook for 5 minutes.
3. Spread the ground beef on a baking pan and cook it in oven or stir-fry until brown.
4. Sprinkle the stir-fry ground beef in the sauce, mix well. Add two cups boiled water, cover and cook it for about 22 minutes.
5. Add to the stew white pepper, salt and cardamom, cook it for about 5 minutes, remove from heat.
6. Serve with injera bread or white rice.

Servings: 3

Ingredients:

- ½ cup quinoa
- 2 table-spoons extra virgin olive oil
- 1 tea-spoon ground cumin
- ¼ tea-spoon red pepper flakes or to taste
- 1 cup water
- Juice of a lime
- ½ tea-spoon salt
- ¾ cup cherry tomatoes, halved
- 3 green onions, finely chopped
- A handful fresh cilantro, chopped
- 7.5 ounces canned black beans, drained, rinsed
- Salt to taste
- Pepper to taste

Method:

1. Pour water into the instant pot. Add quinoa and ½ tea-spoon salt.
2. Close the lid. Select 'Manual' button and set the timer for 1 minute.
3. Let the steam release naturally for about 8 minutes. Then quick release the pressure.
4. Fluff the quinoa with a fork and transfer into a serving bowl.
5. Add rest of the ingredients and toss well.
6. Serve either chilled or at room temperature.

Servings: 6

Ingredients:

- 6 ounces tri-color rotini pasta, cook according to instructions on the package
- 1 small red bell pepper, sliced
- 1 small green bell pepper, sliced
- 6 ounces Italian salami, finely chopped
- 1 medium red onion, chopped
- 3 ounces canned sliced black olives
- 8 table-spoons Italian style salad dressing
- 1 ½ packages (0.7 ounces each) dry Italian style salad dressing mix or to taste
- 4 ounces small fresh mozzarella balls (ciliegine)
- ¼ cup parmesan cheese, shredded

Method:

1. Add all the ingredients except dry salad dressing and Parmesan cheese into a bowl and toss well.
2. Add dry dressing and toss again. Taste and add more dressing if necessary.
3. Sprinkle Parmesan cheese.
4. Chill for a while if desired and serve.

Servings: 1-2

Ingredients:

- 1 table-spoon turmeric
- 1 onion (chopped)
- 1 table-spoon ginger (minced)
- 1 table-spoon garlic (minced)
- ½ cup oil
- 2-3 cup water
- ¾ cup shiro
- salt, to taste

Method:

1. Start with cooking the onions dry in a large pan or wok, stirring frequently, for several minutes on medium-high heat. When the onions have softened, add the oil.
2. When the oil has heated through, add the turmeric and mix well. Boil a few minutes, after add 2 cups of water and take to a boil.
3. Add the shiro slowly and stir briskly (preferably with a whisk) to remove any lumps. Add more oil as needed and continue cooking. Add the ginger and garlic and salt, if desired, and stir.
4. Serve.

Servings:

Ingredients:

- 6 Idaho potatoes, cut into bite size pieces
- 2 ¼ cups carrots, chopped
- 1 ½ cups corn kernels, fresh or frozen
- 3 cups water
- 1 ½ cups green peas, fresh or frozen

For dressing:

- 8 table-spoons vegan mayonnaise
- Himalayan pink salt or salt to taste
- 5 black or green olives, minced
- ¼ tea-spoon pepper powder

Method:

1. Add potatoes and carrots into the instant pot. Pour water in it.
2. Close the lid. Select 'Manual' button on low pressure and set the timer for 12 minutes.
3. When the timer goes off, quick release excess pressure.
4. Add peas and corn and close the lid again.
5. Select 'Manual' button on low pressure and set the timer for 0 minute (zero).
6. When the timer goes off, quick release excess pressure.

Servings: 8-10

Ingredients:

<u>For the dressing:</u>

- 2 cups fresh Italian parsley, loosely packed
- ½ tea-spoon dried oregano
- ½ cup red wine vinegar
- 1 cup extra virgin olive oil
- ½ tea-spoon pepper
- 3 tea-spoons honey
- 20-25 big leaves of basil
- 4 cloves garlic, peeled
- 1 ½ tea-spoon salt or to taste

<u>For salad:</u>

- 2 large heads romaine lettuce, washed, chopped
- ½ cup green olives, pitted
- 2 cups hothouse cucumber, sliced
- 1 cup cherry tomatoes or grape tomatoes, halved
- 2 large bell peppers, chopped
- 2 large carrots, halved, thinly sliced
- 1 cup ricotta

Method:

1. Mixture together all the elements of the salad in a large boule.
2. Add all the ingredients of the dressing into a blender and blend until smooth.
3. Pour about half the dressing over the salad and toss well.
4. Taste and add more dressing if required.

Servings: 4-6

Ingredients:

- a head of cabbage (finely chopped)
- 3 cups of potatoes (chopped)
- 4 cloves garlic (minced)
- 2 medium-large carrots (sliced)
- 2 tea-spoons olive oil
- 2 tea-spoon ginger (minced)
- 1 medium sized onion (chopped)
- 1 tea-spoon turmeric powder
- 1/2 tea-spoon cumin powder
- 1/2 tea-spoon fenugreek seeds
- 1/2 tea-spoon cardamom powder
- 1/2 tea-spoon cinnamon powder
- 1/4 tea-spoon powdered cloves

Method:

1. Start making your atkilt wot by warming the oil in a large skillet, then adding the garlic, onion and ginger.
2. For a little extra heat, consider adding in a chopped green chili at this stage. Cook these for 6 minutes, or until the onions start looking translucent. Add in the flavors and mix up whereas cooking for another 2 minutes.
3. Next, add the carrots, potato and cabbage and mix well, adding a ¼ tea-spoon of salt. Cover and cook for a further 15 minutes, stirring a couple of times to avoid excess browning.
4. Don't add water! The liquid from the vegetables will stay in the pan under the cover and help to keep things nice and moist. Add a little extra salt to taste, along with a generous

amount of black pepper and a little extra oil if you feel it is necessary.

5. Cook until the vegetables are tender.

Servings: 4-6

Ingredients:

- 3 table-spoon oil
- ¾ cup green onions, chopped
- 1 ½ cups rice
- 1 ½ cans (14 ounces each) pinto beans, drained, rinsed
- 1 bay leaf
- 1 ½ pounds smoked sausage, sliced
- 5 cloves garlic, minced
- 3 cups chicken broth
- Salt to taste
- Pepper to taste

Method:

1. Select 'Sauté' button. Add oil. When the oil is heated, add sausage, garlic and green onions and cook until onions are translucent.
2. Add rest of the ingredients and stir. Press 'Cancel' button.
3. Close the lid. 'Select 'Rice' button.
4. When the rice cycle completes, fluff the rice with a fork.

Servings: 4

Ingredients:

- 4 small carrots, halved
- 4 thin asparagus spears, trimmed
- 1 cup broccoli florets or cauliflower florets
- 1 endive, leaves separated
- 2 spring onions, trimmed, halved
- 1 ounce haricot verts, trimmed
- Flaky sea salt to taste
- 4 red radishes, trimmed, thinly sliced
- ½ celery heart, cut into 4 wedges
- 1 small fennel bulbs, halved
- 1 head Little Gem lettuce, leaves separated
- ¼ bunch watercress, tough stem removed
- Lemon juice, as required
- ½ cup olive oil

Method:

1. Decorate all the vegetables on a large serving platter in any manner you desire.
2. Drizzle lemon juice all over. Season with salt.
3. Divide the oil in 4 small bowls, for dipping. Serve salad with oil.

Servings: 2

Ingredients:

- ½ pint mixed cherry tomatoes, preferably heirloom tomatoes, halved
- Flaky sea salt to taste
- 4 ounces buffalo mozzarella or mozzarella cheese, at room temperature, torn into pieces
- A handful small basil leaves
- 3 ½ table-spoons extra-virgin olive oil, divided
- 1 pound mixed medium and large tomatoes, preferably heirloom, thinly sliced or cut into wedges
- Coarsely ground pepper to taste
- Country bread slices, toasted, to serve

Method:

1. Add cherry tomatoes, salt and ½ table-spoon oil into a bowl and toss well.
2. Place tomato slices, slightly overlapping each other on a serving platter. Sprinkle a generous amount of salt.
3. Place mozzarella cheese over the tomatoes. Sprinkle salt over the cheese.
4. Spread the cherry tomatoes over the salad. Drizzle remaining oil. Sprinkle pepper.
5. Set aside for a while for the flavors to set in.
6. Garnish with basil and serve with country bread slices.

Servings: 4

Ingredients:

- 5 table-spoons olive oil
- 4 table-spoons fresh lemon juice
- 2 medium-large tomatoes (peeled and chopped)
- 1 cup (8 oz) green lentil (soaked overnight)
- 1 red onion (finely chopped)
- 1 green chili pepper (seeded and chopped)
- ½ tea-spoon prepared mustard
- Salt & newly milled black pepper to taste

Method:

1. Prepare a saucepan and place the lentils, cover with water and bring to a boil.
2. Simmer for about 50 minutes until soft, drain, then turn into a bowl and mash lightly with a potato masher.
3. Add the remaining ingredients and mix well. Adjust seasonings to taste.
4. Chill before serving.

Servings: 2

Ingredients:

<u>For dressing:</u>

- 2 table-spoons olive oil
- 2 table-spoons finely chopped shallot
- ½ table-spoon fresh oregano, chopped
- 1 table-spoon red wine vinegar
- 1 table-spoon fresh lemon juice
- Salt to taste

<u>For salad:</u>

- 2 ounces local bread, cut into small pieces (about 2 cups)
- 2 table-spoons olive oil
- ½ slight head radicchio, torn into bite size pieces
- ½ cup fresh parsley leaves, chopped
- 1.5 ounces aged sheep milk cheese like Manchego, shaved
- ½ small fennel bulb, thinly sliced
- ¼ cup green olive, pitted, halved
- 1.8 ounces hard salami, thinly sliced
- ½ tea-spoon lemon zest, freshly grated

Method:

1. To make dressing: Add all the ingredients of dressing into a small bowl and whisk well. Cover and set sideways whereas for the flavors to set in.
2. Meanwhile, add bread, lemon zest and 2 table-spoons oil into a bowl and toss well. Sprinkle salt and pepper.
3. Spread on a rimmed baking sheet.
4. Bake in a preheated oven at 400° F for 9-10 minutes or until crisp on the top. Cool completely.
5. Add all the salad ingredients into a bowl and toss well. Add bread and toss well.
6. Pour dressing on top. Toss well.

7. Chill if desired or serve immediately.

Servings: 4

Ingredients:

- 4 tea-spoons vegetable oil
- 2 large cloves garlic, minced
- ½ tea-spoon salt
- 1 carrot, peeled, chopped
- ½ red bell pepper, chopped
- ½ green bell pepper, chopped
- 7 ounces corn kernels
- ¼ cup raisins
- 2 table-spoons golden raisins
- ¼ cup dried cranberries
- 1 table-spoon butter, divided
- 2 cups hot water + extra to soak
- 1 cup basmati rice, rinsed, drained

Method:

1. Add raisins, golden raisins and dried cranberries into a bowl and fill the bowl with hot water. Let it soak for a while.
2. Meanwhile, select 'Sauté' button. Add oil. Once the oil is frenzied, add onion and fry until translucent. Add garlic and cook for about a minute or two until it becomes golden brown.
3. Add rice and salt and cook until the rice is well coated and opaque.
4. Add hot water and stir. Press 'Cancel' button.
5. Close the lid. Select 'Rice' button.
6. Meanwhile, add carrot and bell pepper into a saucepan. Pour enough water to cover. Place saucepan over medium heat. Cook until crisp as well as tender. Drain and set aside.
7. Add corn and ½ table-spoon butter into a microwave safe bowl. Microwave on High for 2-3 minutes.
8. When the rice cycle completes, do not open the lid for a while.

9. Fluff rice with fork.
10. Strain the water of the raisins and add into the rice. Add carrots and corn and mix until well combined.
11. Add ½ table-spoon butter and stir.

Servings: 2

Ingredients:

- ¼ cup dry split yellow peas steep overnight or 2 hours
- ¼ cup dry split green peas steep overnight or 2 hours
- 4-5 garlic cloves (minced)
- 2 tea-spoons ginger (minced)
- 2 tea-spoons oil
- 1 ½ cups water
- ½ red onion (chopped)
- 1/3 tea-spoon turmeric powder
- salt and pepper to taste

Variations:

- Add a 1/2 tea-spoon berbere spice blend for a spicier Wat version
- Add a chopped Serrano pepper.

Method:

1. First, soak the split peas overnight or at least 2 hours in warm water, drain and rinse.
2. In a deep pan, add oil, add onions, ginger and garlic and cook stirring occasionally, until translucent. (add chopped Serrano or Jalapeno if using)
3. Add the turmeric and mix well.
4. Add rinsed split peas, salt, pepper and water. Mix, cover and bring to a boil on medium heat.
5. Reduce heat to low and simmer, partially covered for 40-45 minutes or until peas have softened to your desired consistency. Taste and adjust salt and spice if needed.

6. *Or use a Pressure cooker:* Pressure cook for 1 whistle on high and then on low for 15 minutes. The pictures are of the pressure-cooked stew.
7. Mash the peas if desired. Add some lemon juice if desired and serve. Palates best with a sour flat bread like Injera.

Servings: 8

Ingredients:

- 4 cups frozen cubed hash brown potatoes
- 4 Italian sausage links, cooked, diced
- 12 eggs
- ½ tea-spoon salt
- 4 table-spoons olive oil
- 4 cups cooked ratatouille
- ½ cup milk
- ¼ tea-spoon pepper powder

Method:

1. Place an ovenproof skillet over medium heat.
2. Add oil. When the oil is heated, add hash browns. Cook until brown.
3. Add sausage and ratatouille. Mix well.
4. Add eggs, salt, pepper and milk into a bowl and whisk well.
5. Pour all over the hash brown mixture. Do not stir. Cover with a lid.
6. Lower the heat and cook until it is almost set.
7. Remove the lid of the skillet and broil for a few minutes until it is light brown.

Servings: 2-3

Ingredients:

- 2 pounds collards
- 3 table-spoons ghee or coconut oil
- 3-4 cloves garlic (chopped finely)
- 1 ½ cups water
- 1 table-spoon black cardamom seeds
- 1 table-spoon ground allspice
- 1 table-spoon cumin seeds
- 1 medium-large sweet onion (chopped)
- 1 table-spoon ground clove
- ½ tea-spoon smoked paprika
- ¼ cup rose or white wine vinegar
- 1/8 tea-spoon cayenne
- salt and pepper to taste

Method:

1. Dry toast cardamom, allspice, and cumin in a medium pot for about 2 minutes over low heat. Add ghee and fry 2 minutes more.
2. Add onion and garlic, cooking until soft and slightly translucent.
3. Mixed collards, clove, paprika, cayenne, and water and cook 50-55 minutes over medium heat, until most of the water has evaporated and the collards are completely soft.
4. Top with vinegar, salt and pepper to taste, and serve hot. Enjoy!

Brazilian Rice

Servings: 8

Ingredients:

- ½ cup vegetable oil
- 4 cups water
- 2 cups long grain rice, rinsed
- 2 medium onions, finely chopped
- ½ tea-spoon salt
- 6 cloves garlic, peeled, minced

Method:

1. Boil water.
2. Meanwhile, select 'Sauté' button. Add oil. Once the oil is fiery, add onion and garlic and fry until translucent.
3. Add rice and sauté for 4-5 minutes. Press 'Cancel' button.
4. Pour water and add salt. Stir and close the lid.
5. Select 'Rice' button. When the rice cycle is completed, do not open the lid for 15 minutes.
6. Fluff with a fork and serve.

Servings: 2

Ingredients:

- ¼ cup quick cooking polenta
- 1 ¼ cups water
- 1 ½ table-spoons butter
- 2 eggs
- Toast to serve, as required
- Salt to taste
- Pepper to taste
- 3 table-spoons grated parmesan cheese
- 2 scallions, sliced
- 4 slices pancetta, cooked

Method:

1. Add water and about ¼ tea-spoon water into a saucepan. Place saucepan over medium heat.
2. When it begins to boil, add polenta and whisk well.
3. Reduce heat to medium low. Stir constantly until the mixture thickens.
4. Add cheese and ½ table-spoon butter. Sprinkle salt and pepper and mix well. Turn off the heat.
5. Place a skillet over medium heat. Add remaining butter. When butter melts, add scallions and sauté for 40 seconds.
6. Add eggs, salt and pepper. Do not stir. Let the eggs cook to the consistency you desire.
7. Serve polenta into serving bowls. Place eggs pm top. Place pancetta and serve along with toast.

Yemisir Wot (Berbere Lentils)

Servings: 3-4

Ingredients:

- ¾ cup (185 mL) canola oil
- 1 ½ medium yellow onions (finely chopped)
- ½ cup (125 mL) *berbere spice* (or to taste)
- 1 table-spoon (15 mL) puréed fresh ginger (peeled)
- 2 tea-spoon (10 mL) puréed fresh garlic
- 1 cup dried red lentils
- 3 cups (750 mL) water (plus more if needed)
- ½ tea-spoon (2 mL) fine sea salt (or to taste)

Method:

1. Prepare a medium saucepan and heat oil over medium heat. Add onions. Cook and stir for about 8 minutes.
2. Put in the berbere, ginger and garlic. Cook, stirring, about 2 minutes.
3. Add the lentils. Cook, stirring, 1 minute.
4. Add 3 cups (770 mL) water. Bring to boil over high heat. Reduce heat to medium-low. Simmer, stirring often and adding water if needed, until lentils disintegrate and mixture is a thick stew, about 30 minutes.
5. Taste; season with salt.

Servings: 3

Ingredients:

- 1 medium onion, chopped
- 6 ounces sliced deli ham, finely chopped
- 2 egg whites
- 3 eggs
- ¼ cup mozzarella cheese, shredded
- 1 tea-spoon Italian seasoning
- ¼ tea-spoon pepper powder
- 1 cup cooked angel hair pasta
- ½ table-spoon vegetable oil
- 2 cloves garlic, minced
- 1 table-spoon mozzarella cheese, shredded
- ¼ tea-spoon salt or to taste

Method:

1. Place an ovenproof skillet over medium heat.
2. Add oil. When the oil is heated, add garlic and ham and sauté for a minute.
3. Add egg whites and eggs into a bowl and whisk well. Stir in the cheese, parsley, pepper, salt and Italian seasoning. Add ham and pasta and mix well.
4. Place the skillet back over medium heat. Transfer the pasta mixture into the skillet. Cover with a lid.
5. Cook for 4 minutes. Turn off the heat.
6. Transfer the skillet into an oven.
7. Bake in a preheated oven at 400° F for 14-15 minutes or until set. A toothpick, when inserted in the center, should come out clean.
8. Let it sit for 5 minutes. Slice and serve.

Servings: 3

Ingredients:

- 3 pieces bone-in chicken thighs
- Pepper to taste
- Salt to taste
- 1 ½ table-spoons vegetable oil
- 6 cloves garlic, minced
- 1 ¼ cups rice, rinsed
- ½ tea-spoon turmeric powder
- A handful fresh parsley, chopped, to garnish
- Lime wedges to serve
- 1 table-spoon dried oregano
- 1 small onion, chopped
- 1 cup fresh corn
- 1 ½ cups chicken stock

Method:

1. Select 'Sauté' button. Add oil. When the oil is heated, add chicken and cook until brown.
2. Mixed onion and garlic and fry till brown. Add turmeric and oregano. Sauté for 25-30 seconds.
3. Add rice and corn and sauté for a couple of minutes. Press 'Cancel' button.
4. Pour broth and add the chicken, salt and pepper.
5. Close the lid. Select 'Rice' button. When the rice cycle completes, fluff with a fork.
6. Garnish with parsley and serve with lime wedges.

Servings: 6

Ingredients:

- 1 small zucchini, finely chopped
- ½ cu baby Portobello mushrooms, sliced
- 1 tea-spoon olive oil
- 1 tea-spoon fresh thyme, minced or ¼ tea-spoon dried thyme
- Pepper to taste
- Salt to taste
- 1 package (5.3 ounces) fresh goat's cheese, crumbled
- 3 eggs, lightly beaten
- 1/8 tea-spoon ground nutmeg
- 1 small sweet red pepper, finely chopped
- 1 small red onion, finely chopped
- 2 cloves garlic, minced
- ½ loaf (½ pound) day old French bread, cubed
- 1 cup parmesan cheese, grated
- 1 cup fat free milk

Method:

1. Place a skillet over medium heat. Add oil. When the oil is heated, add zucchini, mushrooms, red pepper and onion. Sauté until slightly soft.
2. Stir in garlic, salt, pepper and thyme. Stir until fragrant.
3. Blubber a baking bowl with a oil.
4. Spread the bread cubes in the baking dish.
5. Layer with bread cubes followed by zucchini – mushroom mixture. Sprinkle goat's cheese and Parmesan cheese.
6. Add eggs, nutmeg and milk into a bowl and whisk well. Pour over the cheese layer.
7. Cover with foil and chill for 6-8 hours.
8. Let it sit on the countertop for 30 minutes before baking.

9. Bake in a preheated oven at 400° F for 14-15 minutes or until set.
10. Let it sit for 5 minutes. Slice and serve preferably with tomato bisque.

Servings: 4-6

Ingredients:

- 1 lb. russet potatoes or 1 lb. white potato (scrubbed, peeled)
- 2 -3 table-spoons grapeseed oil
- 2 table-spoons new flat-leaf Italian sage, chopped
- 1 lemon (juiced, to taste)
- 1/3 cup white onion (finely minced)
- salt and pepper to taste
- 1 green jalapeno pepper, minced (optional)

Method:

1. Start by cutting the potatoes into 2-2 1/2" chunks.
2. Bring a large pot of water to boil and add the potatoes.
3. Cook about 20 minutes or until fork tender.
4. Drain. Colorant potatoes under normal water to stop the cooking procedure.
5. Set aside to cool.
6. In serving bowl combine the oil, white onion, Italian parsley, salt, pepper and jalapeno if using. Add the cooled potatoes, breaking up the chunks into smaller bite sized pieces and tossing with the oil and onion mixture.
7. Refrigerate at least 3.5 hours. Keep chilled until just before serving.
8. Adjust seasonings, adding more lemon juice, etc. if necessary.

Servings: 5

Ingredients:

- 5 chicken thighs, bone-in
- 1 medium onion, chopped into large squares
- 1 table-spoon dried oregano
- 1 can coconut milk
- ½ cup chicken stock
- 2 large red bell peppers, chopped into large squared
- 8-10 whole cloves garlic, peeled
- 3 table-spoons dende oil
- 14 ounces canned diced tomatoes
- Salt to taste
- Pepper to taste

Method:

1. Place red bell pepper, garlic, onion and oregano at the bottom of the instant pot.
2. Place chicken over it. Pour oil, stock and coconut milk over it. Top with tomatoes.
3. Sprinkle salt and pepper liberally over it.
4. Close the lid. Select 'Slow cook' button and set the timer for 2.5 hours or until the chicken is cooked through.
5. Serve over Brazilian rice.

Servings: 3

Ingredients:

- 1 cup onions, chopped
- ½ pound small potatoes, chopped into bite sized pieces
- 4-6 cups kale leaves, discard hard stems and ribs, chopped
- 4 cloves garlic, minced
- 1 can (15 ounces) pinto beans, drained, rinsed
- 4 cups vegetable broth
- ½ tea-spoon dried basil
- ½ tea-spoon dried oregano
- ¼ tea-spoon dried rosemary, crushed or fresh rosemary sprig
- ¼ tea-spoons red pepper flakes
- ¼ tea-spoon fennel seeds
- ¼ cup nondairy milk (optional)
- 1 table-spoon nutritional yeast (optional)

Method:

1. Place a soup pot over medium heat. Add onions and a table-spoon of water and sauté until onions turn soft. Add garlic and sauté for a minute.
2. Add rest of the ingredients except kale, milk and nutritional yeast.
3. When it begins to boil, lower the heat and cover with a lid.
4. Cook until the potatoes are tender.
5. Add kale, cover, and cook for 6-8 minutes until kale turn bright green and tender as well.
6. Remove about half the soup and blend in a blender until smooth and pour it back to the pot.
7. Heat thoroughly. Taste and adjust the seasonings if necessary.
8. Add milk and nutritional yeast. Mix well. Discard rosemary sprig.
9. Ladle into soup bowls and serve.

Servings: 4

Ingredients:

- 4 medium-large potatoes (diced)
- 2 large beets (diced)
- 1 ½ tea-spoons fresh garlic (minced)
- 1 cup water (or more as needed)
- 1 yellow onion (diced)
- ½ tea-spoon salt (divided, or as needed)
- ¼ cup canola oil
- 1 ½ tea-spoons minced fresh ginger (optional)

Method:

1. Prepare a large pot and heat oil over medium heat; add onion and a pinch of salt. Cook and stir onion until softened and translucent, about 8-10 minutes. Add garlic and ginger; fry and stirring till perfumed, about 1 minute.
2. Add beets and stir to combine. Pour water over beet combination and sprinkling ½ tea-spoon salt; bring to a boil.
3. Cover pot and reduce heat to medium-low; simmer, stirring occasionally, until beets are easily pierced with a fork, 20 to 25 minutes. Add potatoes and fry till potatoes are soft but not falling apart, about 15 minutes.
4. Serve with bread or Ethiopian Injera.

Servings:

Ingredients:

- 1.1 pounds carne seca
- 3.5 ounces cream
- 8.8 ounces manioc / yucca
- ¼ cup milk
- Salt to taste
- 1 table-spoon butter
- A handful parsley, chopped
- 1 medium onion, chopped

Method:

1. Place carne seca in a large bowl. Pour enough water to fill the bowl. Let it soak for 24 hours. Drain.
2. Add carne seca into the pressure cooker. Cover with water.
3. Close the lid. Select 'Meat / Stew' button and set the timer for 30 minutes. Let the pressure release naturally.
4. When cooked, drain and place on your cutting board. When calm sufficient to handle, shred with a pair of splits.
5. Place manioc into the pressure cooker. Cover with water.
6. Close the lid. Select 'Manual' button and set the timer for 25 minutes. Let the pressure release naturally.
7. Remove the manioc from the pot and discard the water. Discard the hard fiber from the center and mash the rest. Add into a bowl.
8. Add milk and cream and mix until smooth.
9. Press 'Sauté' button. Add butter. When butter melts, add onions and sauté until it is translucent.
10. Stir in the carne seca, salt and parsley. Cook for 5-6 minutes. Switch off the instant pot.

11. Transfer into a baking dish. Spread it all over the bottom of
    the dish. Spread the manioc mixture evenly over the carne
    seca.
12. Bake in a preheated oven at 390 F until the top is golden
    brown.

Servings: 3

Ingredients:

- 3 vegetarian sausages, sliced
- 5 ounces gnocchi
- 1 carrot, peeled, chopped
- 1 small onion, chopped
- 1 celery rib, chopped
- 2 cups spinach, chopped
- 1 cup mushrooms, sliced
- 10 ounces canned diced tomatoes with Italian seasoning
- 2 cups vegetable broth
- Freshly ground black pepper to taste
- Salt to taste
- ½ tea-spoon Italian seasoning or to taste

To serve:

- Handful fresh parsley, chopped
- Parmesan cheese, grated, as required

Method:

1. Add all the ingredients except spinach and gnocchi into a soup pot. Place the soup pot over medium heat.
2. Cover and cook until the vegetables are nearly tender.
3. Add gnocchi and spinach and cook for a few minutes until done.
4. Ladle into soup bowls. Garnish with Parmesan cheese and parsley and serve.

Servings: 4-6

Ingredients:

- 3 cups chickpea flour
- 2 tea-spoons salt
- 2 table-spoons onions (finely grated)
- 1 tea-spoon garlic (finely chopped)
- 1 tea-spoon white pepper
- ¾ - 1 cup water
- vegetable oil (for frying)

For the sauce:

- 2 cups onions (finely chopped)
- 1 ½ cups water
- 1 tea-spoon salt
- 1 table-spoon garlic (finely chopped)
- ½ cup berbere
- ¼ cup vegetable oil

Method:

1. First, sift the flour, 2 tea-spoons of salt and the white pepper into a deep bowl.
2. Make a well in the center and combine ¾ cup water, the onions and garlic in the well.
3. Slowly stir the dry elements in the water and onions and, when blended, beat vigorously with a spoon or knead with your hands until the dough is smooth and can be gathered into a ball.
4. If the dough crumbles, add up to ¼ cup water, 1 tea-spoon at a time, until the dough comes together.
5. On a lightly floured surface, roll out the dough until it is about ¼ inch thick.

6. With a small sharp knife, cut the dough into fish shapes about 3 inches long and 1 inch wide. If you need, you can use the point of the knife to decorate the top of each "fish" with balances and fins.
7. Pour oil into a deep fryer or a large, heavy saucepan to a depth of 2-3 inches.
8. Heat until it reaches 360 F and fry the "fish" for 3-4 minutes, turning them frequently until they puff slightly and are golden brown.
9. As they brown, transfer them to paper towels to drain.
10. Once you are done the fish you can make the sauce.
11. In a weighty 10-12-inch-wide pan cook the chopped onions for 5-6 minutes until they are soft and dry.
12. Pour in the ¼ cup oil and when it's hot, add the berbere and garlic and stir for a minute.
13. Pour in the 1 ½ cups water and cook until the sauce is slightly thickened.
14. Season with salt and then place the "fish" in the skillet and baste them with the sauce.
15. Lower the heat, cover the pan and simmer for 30 minutes.
16. To serve, arrange the "fish" on a platter and pour the sauce over them.

Servings: 6-8

Ingredients:

- 2 pounds patinho or silverside beef, flattened, cut into 8 strips of 2-3 inches wide
- 2 carrots, peeled, thinly sliced
- 1 onion, sliced
- 8 strips bacon
- 2 tea-spoons dried oregano
- 2 cans (16 ounces each) whole tomatoes with its liquid
- Salt to taste
- 6 tomato cans water

Method:

1. Place the beef strips on your countertop. Place bacon, carrot and onions on the beef strips. Roll and secure with toothpicks.
2. Add tomatoes, water, oregano and salt in the instant pot. Mix well.
3. Place the rolled beef in the cooker. The rolls should be covered with water. If it is not covered, add some more water.
4. Close the lid. Select 'Meat / Stew' button and set the timer for 35 minutes. Once the clock goes off, let the pressure release normally.
5. Select 'Sauté' button and press 'Adjust' button twice. Simmer uncovered until the thickness of the gravy you desire is achieved.
6. Serve with rice, sautéed greens and beans.

Servings: 8

Ingredients:

- 1 large onion, thinly sliced
- 10 table-spoons red wine vinegar
- Salt to taste
- Freshly ground pepper to taste
- ½ pound Genoa salami
- ½ pound deli sliced Capicola
- ½ -1 cup sliced pickled pepperoncini (optional)
- 3 tea-spoons dried oregano
- 2 loaves soft Italian bread (12 inches each)
- 10 table-spoons extra-virgin olive oil
- ½ pound deli sliced provolone cheese
- ½ pound deli sliced boiled ham
- 1 head iceberg lettuce, finely shredded
- ½ pound deli sliced mortadella
- 6 plum tomatoes, thinly sliced

Method:

1. Place onions in a bowl of cold water for about 15 minutes and drain.
2. Halve the bread lengthwise and scoop some bread from the inside of the halved bread.
3. Trickle 2 table-spoons oil on the bottom half of each loaf.
4. Trickle 2 table-spoons vinegar on the bottom half of each loaf.
5. Sprinkle salt and pepper over it.
6. Place cheese and salami over it. Place onions over it. Layer with lettuce followed by pepperoncini and tomatoes.
7. Trickle 3 table-spoons of vinegar and 2 table-spoons olive oil over it. Scatter oregano.
8. Sprinkle salt and pepper.

9. Trickle remaining oil and vinegar on the cut part of the top
    of the loaves.
10. Cover the sandwiches with the top half of the loaves.
11. Cut each sandwich into 4 and serve.

Servings: 2

Ingredients:

- ½ pound salt cod chunks or fillets
- ½ cup extra-virgin olive oil, divided
- Salt to taste
- Pepper to taste
- A handful flat leaf parsley, finely chopped
- Lemon wedges to serve (optional)
- 1 pound medium potatoes
- 1 large onion, sliced
- 1/3 cup kalamata or green or Spanish olives, halved
- 1-2 eggs, hard-boiled, peeled, sliced

Method:

1. Add salt cod into a container with a lid. Cover with water. Close the lid and refrigerate for 24-48 hours. Replace with fresh water every 8-10 hours.
2. Drain and add into the instant pot. Cover with water.
3. Close the lid. Select 'Manual' and set the timer for 5 minutes. Once the clock goes off, quick release extra pressure. Drain the water and place on your cutting board.
4. When cool enough to handle, shred the cod using your hands and make into tiny pieces.
5. Meanwhile, pour 2-3 cups water into the instant pot. Place potatoes in it.
6. Close the lid. Select 'Manual' button and set the timer for 10 minutes. When the timer goes off, let the pressure release naturally for 8 minutes after which quick release excess pressure.
7. Peel the potatoes and slice into ½ inch slices.
8. Drain the water in the pot and wipe clean.

9. Select 'Sauté' button. Add 2 table-spoons oil. When the oil is heated, add onions and sauté until golden brown in color.
10. Add remaining oil, cod, potatoes, salt and pepper and sauté until hot. Switch off the pot.
11. Add olives and parsley. Fold gently. Place egg slices on top. Serve with lemon wedges.

Servings: 2

Ingredients:

<u>For no rise spelt crust:</u>

- ¾ cup warm water
- 4 tea-spoons active yeast
- 2/3 tea-spoon salt
- 1 ½ cups spelt flour
- 4 tea-spoons extra virgin olive oil
- 2 tea-spoons maple syrup
- 2 table-spoons cornstarch or arrowroot starch

<u>For BBQ tofu:</u>

- 4 table-spoons BBQ sauce
- 1 tea-spoon garlic powder or paste
- 5-6 tea-spoons Sriracha sauce or any other hot sauce
- 2 cups firm tofu, pressed, cubed

<u>Other toppings:</u>

- 1 onion, halved, sliced
- Marinara sauce as required
- 1 bell pepper, sliced
- 1 cup almond milk pepper Jack cheese, shredded
- 2 table-spoons cilantro, chopped

Method:

1. For BBQ tofu: Place the tofu in between kitchen towels. Place something heavy over it for 18 minutes.
2. Add tofu, BBQ sauce, Sriracha sauce and garlic into a bowl and mix well. Let it marinate until use.
3. Meanwhile make spelt crust as follows: Add water, yeast and maple syrup into a large bowl and stir. Set aside for 5-7 minutes or until it becomes frothy.

4. Mix together in another bowl, spelt flour, cornstarch and salt.
5. Add the dry ingredient mixture into the frothy mixture. Add oil and knead until you get smooth dough.
6. Divide the dough into 2 equal portions. Shape into balls.
7. Place on a parchment paper and roll the dough into 2 ovals of about 12 inches size. Place on a baking sheet. Leave it at a warm place for about 10 minutes.
8. Spread marinara sauce over the rolled dough. Scatter the onions and peppers over it. Season with salt and pepper.
9. Layer with tofu pieces. Pour the remaining marinade over it. Sprinkle cheese on top.
10. Bake in a preheated oven at 450 ° F for about 12-15 minutes. Remove from oven.
11. Garnish with cilantro and serve.

Servings: 7

Ingredients:

- 2 lb monkfish
- 1 1/2 table-spoons berbere
- salt, to taste
- oil, for frying
- 1 thinly sliced onion
- 2 finely chopped garlic cloves
- 3 finely chopped small chilis
- juice of 1 lime

Method:

1. Start by sprinkling berbere over fish and leave for 1 hour to marinate.
2. Heat enough oil in a large skillet for deep frying. Add fish pieces and cook till golden on all sides and cooked through. Remove to a paper towel lined bowl to absorb extra oil. Sprinkle with a little salt.
3. Add onions and cook until golden and caramelized, about 12 minutes. Most of the oil will have evaporated. Add garlic and chilis. Cook for 1 more minute.
4. Return fish to the pan. Add lime juice and toss to combine.
5. Serve with lime and an extra garnish of more berbere.

Servings: 3

Ingredients:

- ¾ pound large shrimp, cleaned, deveined, with its tail
- 1 ½ table-spoon olive oil, divided
- 1 garlic clove, minced
- 4 table-spoons butter
- 1 ½ cups whole milk
- ¾ cup Catupiry
- Salt to taste
- Black pepper to taste
- 1 small onion, minced
- 2 table-spoons brandy
- 2 table-spoons all-purpose flour
- ¼ tea-spoon nutmeg
- A handful Italian parsley, finely chopped

Method:

1. Rinse the shrimp in a bowl of cold water. Dry the shrimp with a clean towel. Add into a bowl. Sprinkle salt and pepper.
2. Set aside a 3-4 shrimp for garnishing. Discard the tail of the remaining shrimp and add it back into the bowl. Chill for a couple of hours.
3. Select 'Sauté' button. Add ½ table-spoon oil. When the oil is heated, add the 3-4 shrimp that was kept aside. Cook for 2 minutes. Flip sides and cook until pink and the edges are slightly golden. Remove with a slotted spoon and set aside again.
4. Add remaining oil into the instant pot. When the oil is heated, add onion and sauté until translucent.
5. Stir in the garlic and shrimp without tail and cook until pink on both the side.

6. Add brandy and cook until dry. Remove the shrimp and add into another bowl. Scrape any browned bits and add into the bowl.
7. Wipe the pot clean. Add butter. Select 'Sauté' button. When the butter melts, add a table-spoon of flour at a time and stir vigorously until smooth and light golden brown in color.
8. Pour ½ cup milk at a time and whisk constantly all the times. When it begins to boil, add salt, pepper and nutmeg and mix well.
9. Add the shrimp and onion mixture. Taste and adjust the salt if necessary. Press 'Cancel' button.
10. Transfer into a baking dish. Spread Catupiry over the shrimp mixture. Broil for a few minutes in a preheated oven until golden brown.
11. Place the shrimp with tail on top. Sprinkle parsley on top and serve.

Servings: 3-4

Ingredients:

- 12 ounces pasta egg tagliolini or bucatini spaghetti
- Freshly cracked pepper to taste
- 2/3 cup Pecorino, finely grated
- 1 ½ cups Grana Padano or parmesan cheese, finely grated
- 6 table-spoons unsalted butter, cubed, divided
- Kosher salt to taste

Method:

1. Cook the pasta following the instructions on the package but drain the water 2 minutes before the time mentioned on the package. Retain some of the cooked water (about 2 cups).
2. Place a big weighty bottom skillet over average heat. Add 4 table-spoons butter. When butter melts, add pepper and toast lightly.
3. Add about a cup of the retained water. When the water begins to boil, add pasta and 3 table-spoons butter.
4. Lower the heat and add Grana Padano cheese. Stir and toss using tongs. When the cheese melts, turn off the heat.
5. Stir in the Pecorino and toss until the cheese melts completely and the pasta is cooked. Add more of the retained water if the sauce is too thick.
6. Spoon into warmed bowls and serve.

Servings: 2

Ingredients:

- 1 very small red onion, thinly sliced, separated into rings
- 1 small tomato, deseeded, chopped
- ½ table-spoon extra-virgin olive oil
- 1 baguette (8-10 inches long), preferably whole grain
- 1 cup romaine lettuce, shredded
- 7 ounces canned artichoke hearts, rinsed, chopped
- 1 table-spoon balsamic vinegar
- ½ tea-spoon dried oregano
- 1 slice provolone cheese (about 1 ounce), halved
- 1/8 cup sliced pepperoncini (optional)

Method:

1. Add onions rings into a bowl of cold water. Set aside for a while. Drain and dry with paper towels.
2. Add artichoke hearts, oregano, vinegar, tomato and oil into a bowl. Toss until well combined.
3. Halve the baguettes lengthwise into 2 equal portions. Carefully scoop out a little of the bread from each half of the baguette.
4. To serve: Place cheese on the bottom half of the baguette. Place artichoke mixture on it. Spread it evenly.
5. Place onion rings, lettuce and pepperoncini. Cover with the top half of the baguette. Chop into 2 halves and serve.

Servings: 2-3

Ingredients:

- ¾ pound jumbo raw shrimp, peeled, deveined
- 1 clove garlic, minced
- 1 clove garlic, coarsely chopped
- ½ tea-spoon pepper powder, divided
- 1 medium orange or red bell pepper, deseeded, sliced
- 1 medium onion, chopped
- ¼ cup canned diced tomatoes
- A handful fresh parsley or cilantro, chopped + extra to garnish
- 3 table-spoons chicken or vegetable broth
- ½ tea-spoon ground ginger
- 1 ounce cream cheese, softened
- ½ tea-spoon salt, divided
- 1 large leaf basil sliced + extra to garnish
- ½ cup canned coconut milk
- 1 table-spoon lime juice
- ½ tea-spoon sweet paprika (optional)
- ½ red jalapeño pepper, thinly sliced
- 2 ½ table-spoons olive oil or vegetable oil, divided

Method:

1. Add shrimp. Toss with ½ table-spoon oil, minced garlic, ¼ tea-spoon pepper and ¼ tea-spoon salt. Set aside for a while.
2. Press 'Sauté' button. Add 1-table-spoon oil. When the oil is heated, onion and bell pepper and sauté until slightly tender.
3. Add chopped garlic and sauté for a minute. Stir the diced tomatoes, basil and parsley and sauté for a minute. Remove the vegetables and add into a blender.

4. Add coconut milk, broth, ground ginger, salt, pepper, paprika and lime juice into the blender and blend until smooth.
5. Wipe the pot clean and add 1-table-spoon oil. When the oil is heated, add shrimp and cook until pink on both the sides. Remove the shrimp and set aside.
6. Pour the blended mixture into the pot. Press 'Adjust' button twice and simmer until heated thoroughly. Add cream cheese and mix. When cream cheese melts and is well blended in the mixture, add shrimp and mix until well coated.
7. Garnish with basil and parsley and serve over noodles or white rice.

Servings: 2-3

Ingredients:

- ¾ cup dried cannellini beans, soaked in water overnight
- 1 medium carrot, scrubbed, cut into 2 halves crosswise
- ½ head garlic, halved crosswise
- 1 clove garlic, chopped
- 1 small sprig rosemary
- ¼ tea-spoon crushed red pepper flakes + extra for garnishing
- 1 ½ table-spoons olive oil + extra to drizzle
- 7.2 ounces canned peeled whole tomatoes
- 1.5 ounces dried lasagna or any other flat pasta, broken into 1 inch pieces
- ½ parmesan rind (about 1 ounce)
- Shaved parmesan cheese, to serve
- 1 celery stalk, halved crosswise
- 3 sprigs parsley
- 1 bay leaf
- Kosher salt to taste
- Freshly ground pepper to taste
- 1 medium onion, chopped
- 6 table-spoons dry white wine
- ¼ small head escarole, torn into 2 inch pieces
- 1 quart water or more if required

Method:

1. Add Parmesan rind, beans, carrots, ½ head garlic, bay leaves, water, celery, herbs and chilies into a soup pot.
2. Place the pot over medium heat. When the water begins to boil, lower the heat and cover with a lid. Cook until the beans are soft. It may take a couple of hours.

3. Add salt and pepper and stir. Turn off the heat. Let the soup rest for 35 minutes.
4. Remove vegetables, rind and herbs with a slotted spoon and discard.
5. Place a pot over medium heat. Add oil. When the oil is heated, add onions and garlic and sauté until onions are translucent.
6. Crush the tomatoes with your hands and add into the pot. Stir frequently until the liquid in the soup pot is dry.
7. Stir in the wine. Cook until nearly dry.
8. Stir in the beans with the cooked liquid. Simmer until the beans are well blended.
9. Stir in the pasta. Add more water if required. Cook until the pasta is al dente. Add more water if required.
10. Add escarole and cook until it wilts. Add salt and pepper.
11. Divide into soup bowls. Drizzle oil on top. Sprinkle Parmesan cheese and chili flakes on top and serve.

Servings: 4-6

Ingredients:

- 3 medium carrots (peeled)
- 5-6 table-spoons unsalted butter
- ½ tea-spoon ground cardamom
- 1 tea-spoon ground black pepper
- ¼ - ½ tea-spoon cayenne
- 1 shallot (minced)
- 2 garlic cloves (minced)
- Salt to taste
- chives (garnish)
- carrot chips (garnish)

Carrot chips:

- 2-3 thick, medium-large carrots
- salt to taste

Method:

For the carrot chips:

1. Start by preheating your oven to 225° F.
2. You want to use thick (meaning having a large diameter) carrots for the chips because they shrink up a lot during the dehydration process. Slice carrots very thinly into rounds using a mandoline or a very sharp knife.
3. Place carrots on a rack fitted over a baking sheet in a single layer. Sprinkle lightly with salt and bake for an hour to an hour and 18 minutes. They should be relatively crispy at that point, but will crisp even more as they cool. Cool completely before serving.

For the tartare:

1. Bring a medium pot of water up to a boil and season heavily with salt. While the water is coming up, prepare an ice bath (a bowl of cold water with ice). You want to cook the carrots and then shock them in the ice bath to stop the cooking.

2. When the water comes up to a boil, add the carrots and cook until a fork slips easily into the thickest part of the carrot. That can vary contingent on the width — I would say wherever from 6 to 12 minutes. Transfer directly to the snow water to stop the cooking. Remove and dry thoroughly. At this point, you can move fast or save them in the fridge for use a day or two later.

3. If you consume a stand blender with a meat grinder attachment, pass the cooled and dry carrots through the larger, coarse grinding plate. If not, you can use a ricer to realize a ground carrot texture. You don't want sentimentality, so try not to take it too far!

4. Heat the butter in a medium saucepan over medium heat. Add spices and toast for a minute or so until fragrant and nutty. The butter should brown a bit. Add the shallot and garlic and cook another 35 seconds to a minute. Throw in the ground incentives until they are heated through. They should be warm and touchable.

5. Serve warm (you can use a ring mold if you like) and top with chopped chives and carrot chips, if using.

Servings: 3

Ingredients:

- ½ pound dry carioca beans or pinto beans, rinsed
- 3 cups water
- 2 table-spoons olive oil, divided
- ¼ pound thick sliced bacon, chopped
- 3 cloves garlic, minced, divided
- ¾ cup toasted manioc flour
- 2 large eggs
- Salt to taste
- Pepper to taste
- 1 bay leaf
- ½ bunch collard greens, rinsed, dried, thinly sliced
- 7 ounces calabresa sausage, sliced or chorizo or any other smoked sausage
- 1 medium onion, sliced
- 1 green onion, thinly sliced
- A handful fresh parsley, chopped

Method:

1. Add beans to the instant pot along with bay leaf and water.
2. Close the lid. Select 'Beans / Chili' button. When the clock goes off, let the pressure release normally. If the beans are not cooked properly, then add more water if required and cook on 'Manual' option for 8-10 minutes.
3. Drain and set aside.
4. Meanwhile, place a skillet over medium heat. Add 1-table-spoon oil. When the oil is heated, add 2 cloves garlic and sauté until golden brown. Add collard greens and cook until it wilts. Season with salt and pepper and remove into a bowl.
5. Place the skillet back over heat. Add remaining oil. When the oil is heated, add eggs and stir constantly until it is

cooked. Remove the scrambled eggs from the pan and add it into the bowl of collard greens.

6. Press 'Sauté' button and 'Adjust' button once. Add sausage and cook until brown and slightly crisp. Remove the sausage with a located spoon and set sideways. Discard the fat that is remaining in the pot.

7. Add bacon into the pot and cook until crisp. Remove with a slotted spoon and set aside.

8. Add onions and 1 clove garlic into the pot and sauté until translucent.

9. Add the sausage, bacon, collard greens, salt and pepper and mix well. Heat thoroughly.

10. Stir in manioc flour, a little at a time and mix well. The dish should be nice and moist.

11. Transfer into a bowl. Garnish with parsley and spring onions and serve right away.

Servings: 1

Ingredients:

- 1 ½ pounds hanger steak or beef tenderloin (cut into 1/2-inch cubes)
- 6 thin slices navel orange (quartered)
- 3 medium-large ripe tomatoes (chopped) or 1 ½ cups drained, roughly chopped canned tomatoes
- 3 cloves garlic (quartered)
- 2 jalapeños (seeded and thinly sliced)
- 2 red onions (sliced)
- 1 bunch broccolini (in 2-inch pieces)
- 1 table-spoon mild chili powder
- ½ cup unsalted dry-roasted peanuts (coarsely chopped)
- ½ cup dry red wine
- ½ tea-spoon ground cardamom
- ½ tea-spoon ground ginger
- ¼ tea-spoon freshly ground black pepper
- ¼ cup peanut oil
- salt to taste

Method:

1. Start by mixing the chili powder, cardamom, ginger, and pepper in a bowl. Add the beef and toss to coat.
2. Heat the oil in a big skillet on medium-high heat. Add the onions and garlic and fry, rousing constantly, until they begin to brown on the edges. Add the meat, sprinkle it with 1 tea-spoon salt, and stir-fry until it is browned on all sides.
3. Reduce the heat and add the tomatoes, broccolini, jalapeños, peanuts, and wine. Simmer for about a minute,

then season with salt if needed. Cook for about 3 minutes
more.

4. Serve, garnished with orange pieces.

Servings: 4

Ingredients:

- 1-1 ½ kg lamb
- 750 g onion
- 125 ml olive oil
- 2 cloves of garlic
- 2 cm piece of ginger
- 2 table-spoons berbere
- 1 tea-spoon salt
- ½ tea-spoon black pepper
- 1 can (400g) tomato

Method:

1. First, chop the onion finely (in a food processor).
2. Bring water (about 750ml) to a boil.
3. Add the onion to a large pot and cook. Shelter the onion with a lid and stir frequently safeguarding that the onion does not burn.
4. Only when necessary add a little water to stop the onion from burning.
5. When the onion is soft and translucent add the oil (after about 10-15 minutes).
6. Cook 10 minutes until golden
7. Add the berbere and cook on the lowest heat for about 30 minutes stirring once in a while. Only when the onions begin to stick, add a few drops of water.
8. Add the canned tomato.
9. Cut the meat into small bite size pieces.
10. Add the lam to the onion.
11. Press garlic and ginger through a garlic press into the pot.

12. Cook the meat, stirring regularly until the meat is just cooked. They approximately the sauce is complete when oil rises to surface. (Depending on the meat this takes about 10 -30 minutes.) When the sauce thickens (after about 10 minutes) add about 250ml-500ml boiling water. You are observing for a thick and sleek stew.
13. Season with salt and pepper.
14. Serve with Injera bread.

Servings: 8

Ingredients:

- 4 large potatoes, peeled, diced
- 2.2 pounds fresh tomatoes, chopped
- ½ cup garlic, grated
- 2 table-spoons cayenne pepper
- Salt to taste
- Pepper to taste
- 2 large onions, peeled, diced
- 4 table-spoons olive oil
- 2 table-spoons fresh rosemary
- 6 table-spoons fresh thyme

Method:

1. Pour 2 cups water in the instant pot. Place the steamer basket in it. Place the potatoes in the steamer basket. Sprinkle half the garlic over the potatoes. Season with salt and pepper.
2. Close the lid. Select 'Steam' button and set the timer for 25 minutes.
3. When the timer goes off, quick release excess pressure.
4. Remove the steamer basket with the potatoes from the instant pot and discard the water.
5. Press 'Sauté' button. Add onion, tomatoes, olive oil and garlic, most of the herbs, salt, pepper and cayenne pepper into the instant pot.
6. Stir frequently and cook until tomatoes are soft. Blend most of the tomatoes with an immersion blender until nearly smooth.
7. Add the potatoes back into the pot and mix well. Simmer for a couple of minutes.
8. Garnish with remaining herbs and serve.

Servings: 4

Ingredients:

- 10-ounce Collard Greens/Kale (chopped)
- 3 or more table-spoons Niter Ethiopian Spiced Butter or cooking oil
- 2 tea-spoon garlic (minced)
- 1-2 fresh chili pepper or ½ tea-spoon cayenne pepper or more
- 1 ½ tea-spoon ginger (minced)
- 1 large white onion (chopped)
- 1 tea-spoon smoke paprika
- 1 tea-spoon coriander/cumin
- 1 fresh lemon
- ½ tea-spoon cardamom spice

Method:

1. In a large skillet, add oil, spiced butter, garlic, ginger, chili pepper, cumin, cardamom, paprika, sauté for about 30 seconds or more, be careful not to let the ingredients burn.
2. Then add onions, mix with the spices. Sauté for about 3-5
3. Throw in chopped collards, cayenne pepper, lemon juice, continue cooking for another 8-10 minutes until flavors have blend and greens are cooked, according to preference. Adjust seasonings –Salt and pepper, turn off the heat.
4. Remove from the heat and let it cool.
5. Serve with Injera.

Servings: 4

Ingredients:

- 1 smoked ham hock, 3 ounces each
- ½ pound dried black beans, rinsed, soaked in water overnight, drained
- 1 bay leaf

For sofrito:

- 1 medium white onion, chopped
- 1/3 bunch parsley, finely chopped (only leaves)
- 1 table-spoon extra-virgin olive oil
- 2 cloves garlic, chopped
- Kosher salt to taste
- Freshly cracked pepper to taste

Method:

1. Add beans to the instant pot along with bay leaf, ham hock and 3 cups water.
2. Close the lid. Select 'Beans / Chili' button. Once the clock goes off, let the pressure release normally. If the beans are not cooked properly, then add more water if required and cook on 'Manual' option for 8-10 minutes.
3. Transfer into a bowl and set aside.
4. For sofrito: Wipe the pot clean. Select 'Sauté' button. Add oil. When the oil is heated, add onion, garlic and parsley and sauté until translucent. Season with salt and pepper. Add the cooked beans along with water into the pot.
5. Press 'Adjust' button twice and simmer until the mixture is slightly thick. Stir occasionally.

Servings: 2

Ingredients:

- 1 lb. yellow potatoes
- 3 medium carrots (loose)
- 3 table-spoons extra virgin olive oil
- 3 cups water
- 3 cloves garlic
- 2 cups green cabbage
- 2 pieces naan
- 1 ½ tea-spoon berbere spice
- 1 lime
- 1 yellow onions
- ½-inch piece ginger
- ¾ cup green lentils
- salt and pepper to taste

Method:

Prepare the Ingredients:

1. Dice the onion. Mince the garlic and ginger.
2. Rinse the lentils in a fine sieve. Cut the lime in half.
3. Rinse the carrots and cut them into ¼-inch thick coins.
4. Rinse and scrub the potatoes, and cut them into ½-inch cubes.
5. Rinse and dice the cabbage.

Make the Atakilt Wat:

1. Heat 2 table-spoons olive oil in a large pot over medium heat.
2. Add the onion, garlic, ginger and Ethiopian spice mix, and cook until tender and fragrant, about 2-3 minutes.

3. Stir in the carrots, potatoes, cabbage, 1 cup of water and salt and pepper to taste.
4. Bring to simmer and cook for 10 minutes, stirring halfway through.
5. Add the lentils and 2 cups of water. Continue to simmer until the lentils and potatoes are tender, about another 16 minutes, stirring halfway through.

Toast the Naan:

1. When the Atakilt Wat is almost ready, heat 1 tbsp. olive oil in a big pan over average warmth.
2. Add a piece of naan and cook until toasted, about 1 minute per side. Repeat with the second piece of naan.
3. Cut the naan into wedges, if desired.

Bring It All Together:

1. Evenly divide the Atakilt Wat between two bowls.
2. Squeeze the lime juice on top and serve with toasted naan.

Servings: 3

Ingredients:

- 1 cup dried carioca or pinto beans, rinsed, soaked in water overnight
- 1 bay leaf
- 1 small onion, chopped
- Salt to taste
- 4 cups water
- 1 ½ strips bacon, chopped
- 2 cloves garlic, minced

Method:

1. Press 'Sauté' button. Add bacon and cook until brown. Add onion and garlic and sauté until onion turns translucent.
2. Add beans, bay leaf, 5 cups water and stir. Press 'Cancel' button.
3. Close the lid. Select 'Beans / Chili' button. Once the clock goes off, let the pressure release normally.
4. Mash a little of the beans with the back of a spoon. Add salt and stir.
5. Press 'Sauté' button. Press 'Adjust' button twice. Simmer for a while until slightly thick.
6. Discard the bay leaf.
7. Serve over rice.

Servings: 2-3

Ingredients:

- 6 cups vegetable broth
- 6 garlic cloves (minced)
- 2 cups dried yellow split peas
- 2 small onions (diced)
- 1 tea-spoon turmeric
- ½ - 1 tea-spoon *berbere spice* (or to taste)
- ½ tea-spoon mild curry powder
- ½ tea-spoon ground ginger
- ½ tea-spoon garam masala
- salt and pepper to taste

Method:

1. In a pot, bring the 6 cups veggie broth to a boil and add the split peas, then cover and reduce heat to low. Simmer for 30 minutes.
2. While the split peas are simmering, sauté onions and garlic in a nonstick skillet until onions are translucent. Add flavors and carefully mix to coat the onion.
3. Add onion mixture to split peas and simmer for 6 minutes, stirring and scraping the peas to keep them from sticking to the bottom of the pan.
4. Taste and add another ⅛ - ¼ tsp Berbere' if desired. Salt and pepper to taste.

Servings: 8

Ingredients:

- 2 cups brown rice, rinsed
- 2 table-spoons olive oil
- 4 cloves garlic, minced
- 2 stalks celery, finely chopped
- 1 large onion, chopped
- 2 large carrots, finely chopped
- 4 cups low sodium chicken stock
- 2 tea-spoons dried oregano or 2 table-spoons fresh oregano, chopped
- A handful fresh parsley, chopped
- 2 cans (15 ounces each) low sodium black beans, drained, rinsed
- 2 tea-spoons ground cumin
- Salt to taste
- 1 tea-spoon dried chili flakes

Method:

1. Add rice, salt, chili flakes and broth into the instant pot. Stir.
2. Close the lid. Select 'Rice' button.
3. When the rice cycle completes, place a skillet over medium-high heat. Add oil. Once the oil is heated, add onions and fry until translucent. Add garlic and sauté until fragrant.
4. Add all the vegetables and cumin powder and sauté until crisp as well as tender.
5. Add black beans and toss well. Heat thoroughly. Turn off the heat.
6. Fluff the rice with a fork. Transfer the vegetable mixture into it. Mix well.
7. Sprinkle parsley on top and serve.

Servings: 8

Ingredients:

- 8 chicken breast halves, skinless, boneless,
- 2 onions, chopped
- 4 jalapeño peppers, deseeded, chopped
- 6 tomatoes, deseeded, chopped
- 2 bunches fresh parsley, chopped
- 2 table-spoons fresh ginger, minced
- 4 cloves garlic, minced
- 2 cans light coconut milk
- 2 tea-spoons ground cumin
- 2 tea-spoons ground turmeric
- 2 tea-spoons ground cayenne pepper
- 2 tea-spoons ground coriander
- Salt to taste
- 4 table-spoons olive oil
- Pepper to taste

Method:

1. Add all the spices in a bowl. Sprinkle salt and pepper over the chicken and rub with the mixture of spices.
2. Select 'Sauté' button. Add 2 table-spoons oil. When the oil is heated, add chicken and cook until brown on both the sides. Remove with a slotted spoon and set aside.
3. Add remaining oil into the instant pot. When the oil is heated, add ginger, garlic and jalapeño peppers and sauté until the onions turn translucent.
4. Add tomatoes and sauté until slightly soft.
5. Add chicken and coconut milk and stir. Press 'Cancel' button.
6. Close the lid. Select 'Poultry' button and set the timer for 13 minutes.
7. When done, stir and serve garnished with parsley.

Servings: 2-3

Ingredients:

- white fillet fish
- 2 tea-spoons of Mitmita
- 8 tea-spoons of white plain flour
- ½ cup of fine breadcrumbs
- 1 tea-spoon of turmeric
- 1 medium egg
- cooking oil
- salt and pepper (to taste)

Method:

1. Mix the flour and Mitmita, salt and pepper together and set aside.
2. Beat one egg and set aside.
3. Mix the breadcrumbs with the Turmeric and set aside.
4. Now that you have 3 separate items simply, coat the fish in the flour then the egg then the breadcrumbs.
5. Make sure at all 3 stages a good coating is made to your fish.
6. Heat 2cm of cooking oil (you can use corn or sunflower if you like) in a skillet.
7. Now place the breaded fish in the oil and cook for 4 mins on each side or until a deep golden brown.
8. Now place the fish on paper towels to remove any oil and serve.

Servings: 8-10

Ingredients:

- ¾ pound peppered bacon, diced
- 3 pounds collard greens, rinsed, stemmed, torn into pieces
- 1 ½ tea-spoons cayenne pepper
- 1 large onion, chopped
- 1 ½ cups chicken stock
- 3 table-spoons red wine vinegar

Method:

1. Select 'Sauté' button. Add bacon and cook until brown.
2. Add onions and sauté until translucent. Stir in the collard greens. Add chicken stock and pepper. Stir and close the lid. Press 'Cancel' button.
3. Select 'Slow cook' button and set the timer for 1-½ hours.
4. Add red wine vinegar during the last 35 minutes of cooking.
5. If there is too much liquid in the pot, then simmer for a while.

Servings: 4

Ingredients:

- 3 pounds potatoes (peeled and washed)
- 2 eggs (beaten)
- 2 onions (finely chopped)
- Salt & pepper, to taste
- 3 table-spoons olive oil
- Applesauce, for serving

Method:

1. Grate the potatoes using a box grater and place it in cheesecloth. Strain the grated potatoes and remove liquid as much as possible.
2. Take a bowl and place the onion in it. Add the grated potato, beaten eggs, salt and pepper to the bowl.
3. Mix well until the contents are blended well to form a dough-like consistency.
4. Heat the oil in a frying pan over medium-high heat. Using a small ladle, spoon the mixture and flatten it a bit.
5. Place it on the hot oil and fry until golden brown. Flip it to the other side and continue frying until crispy and brown.
6. Transfer to a plate and serve hot with applesauce.

Servings: 8

Ingredients:

- 6 table-spoons olive oil, divided
- 6 cups mushrooms, sliced
- 4 chicken breasts, skinless, thinly sliced
- 2 cans (14.5 ounces each) stewed tomatoes
- 2 onions, thinly sliced
- 4 cloves garlic, crushed
- Salt to taste
- Pepper to taste
- 2 cans (7.6 ounces each) table cream

Method:

1. Select 'Sauté' button. Add 4 table-spoons oil. Once the oil is heated, add onions and cook until onions are translucent.
2. Stir in the garlic and mushrooms and sauté until slightly tender.
3. Transfer the mushrooms into a bowl.
4. Wipe the pot clean. Add 2 table-spoons oil. When the oil is heated, add chicken and cook until golden brown on both the sides.
5. Blend the tomatoes and add into the pot. Also add mushrooms, salt and pepper. Press 'Cancel' button.
6. Press 'Poultry' button and set the timer for 7 minutes.
7. When the timer goes off, quick release excess pressure. Add table cream.
8. Press 'Sauté' button and 'Adjust' button twice. Simmer for 4-5 minutes.
9. Serve hot.

Conclusion

We have come to the end of the book. Thank you for reading and congratulations for reading until the end. I hope you found the book informative and interesting.

This lunch recipe book is definitely one of the most loved, delicious, rich and healthy cook book from across the world.

The recipes often call for fresh herbs, vegetables and fruit. However, these can be replaced with frozen and canned foods as well. It is also possible to change and replace certain ingredients if you don't like them or if they are not available. You can take a judgment call on the same and replace certain ingredients to improve the texture or flavor of the dish.

Modify and experiment with these recipes and create your very own personalized recipes. Do not let cooking become a chore. Rather, make it a fun activity. The recipes in this book are simple, easy to make and delicious. All the recipes have been tested and tasted so the end result will leave you satisfied.

Finally, if you enjoyed this book then I'd like to ask you for a favor. Will you be kind enough to leave a review for this book on Amazon? It would be greatly appreciated!

Thank you and good luck!

9 798609 281463